T0337399

A Shot of Justice

A Shot of Justice
Priority-Setting for Addressing Child Mortality

ALI MEHDI

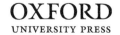

OXFORD
UNIVERSITY PRESS

OXFORD
UNIVERSITY PRESS

Oxford University Press is a department of the University of Oxford.
It furthers the University's objective of excellence in research, scholarship,
and education by publishing worldwide. Oxford is a registered trademark of
Oxford University Press in the UK and in certain other countries.

Published in India by
Oxford University Press
2/11 Ground Floor, Ansari Road, Daryaganj, New Delhi 110 002, India

ISBN-13: 978-0-19-949059-2
ISBN-10: 0-19-949059-7

Typeset in Dante MT Std 10.5/13
by Tranistics Data Technologies, Kolkata 700 091
Printed in India by Nutech Print Services India

Now is the time to make justice a reality for all of God's children
'I have a dream', Martin Luther King, Jr. (1963)

Contents

Tables and Figures

Tables

Figures

Foreword

Public policy and political philosophy rarely go together. This was not always the case. Some of the most well-known names in economics, the discipline most directly involved with the world of policymaking, have also been among the most celebrated political philosophers of the modern era—Adam Smith, Karl Marx, John Maynard Keynes, Friedrich Hayek, to name a few. Despite all our progress and prosperity in the recent past, the dramatic rise in aspirations of our young population has forced policymakers to focus on immediate challenges. They have hardly had the time for political philosophy and its impact on public policy. As a result, the world of policymaking has come to be increasingly dominated by technocrats, characterized by a strong preference for quick solutions with measurable outcomes and, by implication, a limited concern for human complexity and diversity.

One of the worst victims of this disconnect has been children's welfare. Children hold the key to the kind of society that we wish to create in the future and to addressing issues of intergenerational equity. By focusing on children, we may succeed in enforcing the implicit social contract, generating social solidarity, and thereby minimizing societal fragility which has become a pervasive feature of our world.

Several of the targets enshrined in the Sustainable Development Goals (SDGs) are promising from this perspective, and countries should act swiftly to achieve them. Nevertheless, they are not going to be enough. Beyond bare survival through shots of immunization (SDG target 3.2), for instance, our children need a shot of justice. This book is about how public policy can do so in the light of discussions in political philosophy since the publication of John Rawls' path-breaking work, *A Theory of Justice*, in 1971. The author has tackled the complex subject most lucidly and in a style that makes the argument accessible to the common reader. This perhaps reflects his deeply held belief that the challenge of child survival in general, and that of child mortality in particular, concerns not only policymakers and the medical fraternity, but the society at large.

Justice is a highly emotive issue in our part of the world. India has had one of the longest-standing affirmative action policies. Despite the rare consistency with which they have been pursued, their focus has remained more or less immediate, with little focus on the next generation and future of inequality in the country. In the evolving globalizing context, it is important to analyse the potential directions that the patterns of inequality might take and our societal response to the emerging trends, in order to ensure a more equitable future for our children.

For all those concerned about justice and equity, the future of our society, and about children, this book is a must-read. The author—whom I have known even prior to his starting the research that has culminated in this worthy volume—combines extensive data on child survival with highly intensive arguments on the metrics of equality. He has drawn on political philosophy for reaching conclusions that could have wide-ranging implications for the pursuit of justice and equality in public policy. This combination of empirical evidence with the philosophical is rare, commendable and exemplary. I feel that we need more people like him in the world of policymaking who are empirically rooted but also carefully and skillfully use the evidence to test existing philosophical paradigms. This permits him to offer better insights into the existing phenomenon, thereby holding out hope for the next generation. I congratulate him, wish him the best and look forward to reading many such books from him.

Rajiv Kumar
Vice Chairman
NITI Aayog
Government of India
6 July 2018

Preface

This book discusses child survival as a problem of justice. A preventable child death is the worst form of injustice since it implies the violation of one of the most basic human rights—the right to life—and premature curtailment of opportunities that every individual is entitled to. The enormous inequalities that children are born into make a mockery of the promise of equality that every decent society on the planet promises. They are unjust and unacceptable because children who are victims of them cannot be held responsible for them. These inequalities are widening as we make progress in various aspects of life—such as education and health—in both developing and developed countries. In a rapidly developing country like India, where premature mortality has been the world's highest for decades and the general level of education of the masses leaves much to be desired, there are children who have had access to world-class healthcare and education, and are able to compete at the global level. Thankfully, the number of such children has been on the rise, especially following India's liberalization in 1991. It has also raised the general level of aspirations and problematized traditional inequalities of gender, caste, etc., in several parts of the country. Inequality, in this sense, also has the potential of raising the overall threshold and making the pursuit of equality upwardly.

Each and every child in the world deserves the opportunity to excel, to realize his optimal potential. A less unjust society is only possible when inequalities are addressed at the earliest levels—at the level of children. First and foremost, we have to make our societies fairer for children—they should have the first claim on welfare. We need a social contract to maximize opportunities for all children—all of them are the future of our society. The question is—how do we treat our children equally? This book discusses what equality and justice mean in the specific context of children. While doing so, it establishes the practical relevance of modern theories of justice—which have lost 'touch with the reality of contemporary societies' (Habermas 1996: 43)—particularly those presented by two of the greatest political philosophers of the late twentieth century, John Rawls and Amartya Sen. As such, this book is distinctive in more ways than one—

1. It broadens the concern with the persistent problem of child mortality by framing it as a case of injustice, and not simply a technical issue of biomedical concern, with shots of vaccinations as the ultimate solution.

2. It provides a robust theoretical framework for the analysis of child survival and related policies from an equity and efficiency perspective, but also for prioritization and resource allocation in the context of child survival.

3. It represents an opportunity for major theories of justice to engage with the real world, not only to explore real-life implications of their theoretical constructs, but also to make a contribution to policies that impact the lives of people suffering from actual injustices in their worst forms.

4. It puts forth an approach which can be replicated for the analysis of other cases of injustice and policies to tackle them—for instance, caste discrimination and policies of affirmative action in the Indian context and elsewhere.

Analysing historical trends in child survival and its determinants among selected groups in India, it argues that Amartya Sen's approach to justice—which is against absolute priority to any unifocal criterion, and favours a multifocal variable that includes a central focus on the 'maximal potentials' of individuals and is simultaneously sensitive to fairness in procedures and outcomes—seems more plausible than its counterparts from the perspective of child survival. It allows for considerations of equity to be met without necessarily sacrificing the potentials of the better off in terms of access to opportunities and outcomes, and is sensitive to aggregative concerns as well. Justice is not about jealousy against the better off. Such an approach to justice is relevant for affirmative action policies that have long been a source of resentment among historically better off groups around the world, especially in two of the world's largest and most vibrant democracies—India and the US. A first of its kind—as far as its multidisciplinary nature and approach is concerned—this book will be of interest to all those who care about justice and children. It would be of academic relevance to scholars and students of political philosophy, development economics, bioethics, public health, demography, social and medical sciences, specifically those interested in priority setting in public policy from equity and efficiency perspectives. Policymakers and nongovernmental organizations concerned with issues of child survival, human development and early human capital formation or with justice and inequality in basic opportunities, more broadly, would find it stimulating. A lot of data has been presented and analysed, but it has been done in a way that lay readers, not necessarily familiar with the subject, may also be able to follow the arguments being developed through them.

Reference

Habermas, Jürgen. 1996. *Between Facts and Norms*. Cambridge, MA: The MIT Press.

Acknowledgements

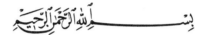

During the decade that I have spent in developing this book, I have accumulated intellectual debt from a wide range of people, and I would like to acknowledge some of them in particular. The late Professor Hermann Schwengel, Prorektor (Research) at the University of Freiburg (Germany), Boike Rehbein, Professor of Society and Transformation in Asia and Africa at the Humboldt University in Berlin (Germany), and Roger Jeffery, Professor of Sociology of South Asia and Associate Director at the Edinburgh India Institute, University of Edinburgh (UK) deserve special gratitude for their patient guidance and supervision, especially during formative years of this work. Rajiv Kumar, my mentor and previous boss at the Indian Council for Research on International Economic Relations (ICRIER), New Delhi and now the Vice Chairman of NITI Aayog, the premier policy think tank of the Government of India, was the prime motivator for my doctoral research and the work in this book that was pursued as part of it. I have always been proud to have him as a mentor, and I have discussed several issues with him over more than a decade of association with him. I hope I finally have a work which can make him feel proud of me. Divya Chaudhry, my colleague at ICRIER, provided enormous help with the data work and other logistics related to putting this book together, and I seriously cannot thank her enough for all her time and contributions. No academic work is possible without inner peace, and I therefore owe a great deal of gratitude to my wife, Mubashira Zaidi, and son, Zaky Zaidi, for their exemplary patience, particularly over several weekends, when families like to spend time outside their homes.

I began with the Name of Allah, the Most Gracious, the Most Merciful because I believe He is the ultimate source of ideas. Let me end here with an anonymous Urdu couplet as a tribute to Him—

Safar to maine kiya tha
Warna saaz-o-saaman uskey they

Main to bus raazdar tha uska
Warna to saarey raaz uskey they

I was the one who travelled
Although all the resources were His

I was only His secret-keeper
Although all secrets were His

Abbreviations

AHS	Annual Health Surveys
AKDN	Agha Khan Development Network
ANC	Antenatal care
ARI	Acute respiratory infection
AWC	Anganwadi center
BCG	Bacillus Calmette–Guérin
BIMARU states	Bihar, Madhya Pradesh, Rajasthan, and Uttar Pradesh
CGHS	Central Government Health Scheme
CRC	Convention on the Rights of the Child
CSDH	Commission on Social Determinants of Health
DHS	Demographic and Health Surveys
DPT	Diphtheria, Pertussis, and Tetanus
EAG	Empowered Action Group
ECD	Early child development
GDP	Gross domestic product
GoI	Government of India
HDI	Human Development Index
ICDS	Integrated Child Development Services
IGME	Inter-agency Group for Child Mortality Estimation
IHDC	India Human Development Survey
IMPAC	Integrated Management of Pregnancy and Childbirth
IMR	Infant mortality rate
LEB	Life expectancy at birth
MDG	Millennium Development Goal

MHA	Ministry of Home Affairs
MoHFW	Ministry of Health and Family Welfare
MoWCD	Ministry of Women and Child Development
MPI	Multidimensional Poverty Index
NCAER	National Council of Applied Economic Research
NCC	National Charter for Children
NCD	Non-communicable disease
NFHS	National Family Health Survey
NHP	National Health Policy
NNMR	Neonatal mortality rate
NPC	National Policy for Children
NSS	National Sample Surveys
OBC	Other backward classes
OECD	Organisation for Economic Co-operation and Development
OPHI	Oxford Poverty and Human Development Initiative
ORS	Oral rehydration solution
PNC	Postnatal care
RCH	Reproductive and Child Health
RGI	Registrar General of India
SC	Scheduled Caste
SDG	Sustainable Development Goal
SRS	Sample Registration System
ST	Scheduled Tribe
TFR	Total fertility rate
U5MR	Under-five mortality rate
UC	Upper caste
UNDP	United Nations Development Programme
UNICEF	United Nations International Children's Emergency Fund
UP	Uttar Pradesh
UT	Union territorie
WDI	World Development Indicator
WHO	World Health Organization

Need for a Shot of Justice

A backlash against the politics and practice of social justice has been brewing in two of the world's largest democracies—India and the US. Both these countries have had a long history of affirmative action policies aimed at addressing inequality of opportunities and outcomes among historically discriminated groups. Such policies have been viewed as unjust and led to a strong sense of neglect, betrayal, and resentment among members of groups considered responsible for historical injustices, predisposing them towards a majoritarian brand of ethno-nationalism that assigns absolute priority to national pride and aggregative development, while perceiving the pursuit of equality and justice for the weaker sections as unjustified appeasement for vote-bank politics. Ironically, such policies have, in several instances, principally benefited a select set of individuals—failing to make much of a difference to the lives of the worst-off members—among target groups, let alone the worse-off among those regarded as historically privileged.

This has led to a legitimate question of the grounds on which justice should be pursued. Justice is a highly complex and dynamic concern, given multiple, overlapping patterns of injustice, evolving over time. It is also contextual—victims of injustice in one context might not be so in another, or worse, be perpetrators. However, ignoring such complexities of injustice, governments have often indulged in the politics of *social* justice, crudely favouring certain groups and excluding others from their pursuit of justice, leading to a backlash not just against the politics and practice, but the very idea, of justice and equality, without them being seriously discussed in public and policy discourse. Both the lack of, as well as the backlash against, equality and justice are making large parts of the world fragile, given the pervasive sense of injustice on both sides. A complex understanding and pursuit of equality and justice have become central for global development, peace, and stability.

There has been a proactive debate in political philosophy on the issue of the *equalisandum*—what is to be equalized across individuals in a just society—since the publication of John Rawls's path-breaking *A Theory of Justice* in 1971, and a number of very influential metrics of justice have been presented based on which proposals and evaluations of equality and justice could be made. There is a need to revisit this debate in the midst of prevailing confusion and disillusionment with justice, particularly in the Indian context. This book is an attempt in this direction. Although social justice has long been an issue of intense political, social, and economic contention in India, there has been little normative literature on the subject,[1] let alone critical engagement with the rich post-Rawlsian Anglo-American literature, with a few exceptions, most notably Amartya Sen's. On the other hand, political philosophers need to take their share of the blame—they have stayed away from the messy world of injustice as well as public and policy debates on the idea of justice—once again, with the limited exception of Sen in the Indian context. One of the concerns of this book is the implications that mundane injustices have for existing theorization on justice, particularly on equalisandum.

Small children are most vulnerable to injustice since they are dependent, and can neither decide for nor defend themselves. At the same time, their welfare is of utmost concern, given that they are the future of households, societies, and nations. Yet, they have not been regarded as subjects of justice, either by parents, policymakers or political philosophers, despite massive intergenerational inequalities which children are born into, which not only influence their life-chances as they grow, but also their very survival in developing countries like India—in their

---

[1] However, there has been an extremely rich body of sociological and social anthropological literature in India on the dynamics of caste, class, and gender, and, to some degree, religion. However, being strongly empirical in focus, it has largely stayed away from normative–theoretical discussions of justice—the work of André Béteille being a notable exception.

first few days, months, and years of birth. What we owe our children is a question all those interested in the future of their households, societies, and nations should ask themselves. Injustice faced by children is the biggest blot on the promise of equality of opportunity—millions of them continue to lack the opportunity to even survive within the first five years of birth. *What does justice mean in the case of children?*

As part of an emerging body of literature on children and justice, the present book tries to address this specific question in the light of the equalisandum debate in political philosophy since Rawls, both conceptually as well as in the context of child survival among selected groups in India—a country with the highest levels of child and premature adult mortality in the world, which is unsurprising given the complex and comprehensive inefficiencies and injustices that characterize Indian society, polity, and the economy. We focus on Sen's metric of justice (capabilities) in particular—while discussing the relevance of others— because, given its multifocal orientation, it is complex and comprehensive in its promise, and seems most promising to analyse and address injustice as it pertains to children. Despite being contextualized in Indian data, the book offers several lessons for the general pursuit of justice as well as for normative discussions of equalisandum in political philosophy. It not only offers an opportunity for theories of justice to engage with, and make a possible contribution to, the real world of injustice, but also highlights the significance of sound principles—and not just sound evidence, as technocrats would have us believe—for the design and assessment of fair and inclusive public policy. As such, the present book is also a humble attempt to raise the bar of public policy discourse beyond the mundane moorings in which it appears to be terribly trapped.

Given the unusual focus and approach of this book, there are bound to be several questions in the minds of its readers. The remainder of the introduction is, thus, dedicated to addressing some of the most prominent ones that could be visualized. For instance: (*a*) why should we focus on survival in discussions of justice; (*b*) why is child mortality an instance of injustice; and (*c*) why do we need to delve into formal theories of justice in this context when neither political philosophers nor policymakers have been interested in each other's domains? The rest of the book is organized in this manner. Chapter 2 discusses the suitability of the prominent metrics of justice in normative terms, with a focus on Sen's capability approach. Chapter 3 presents and analyses data on child survival at international, inter-state and inter-group levels, while Chapter 4 examines the conceptual and empirical architecture of the determinants of child survival—structural (political, economic, social structures), intermediate (community, social/household status), and immediate (modern biomedical healthcare). Finally, grounded in realities of child survival and access to its determinants in the Indian context, Chapter 5 analyses which shot of justice is the most appropriate for the specific case of children, including an assessment of India's child and health policies and brief discussion of the implications of our discussions for political philosophy and affirmative action policies.

Need for Survival

Our struggle for justice begins at birth. Most of us have directly witnessed the massive inequities that children are born into, and which go on to influence—if not completely determine—their lives ahead. The challenge of survival in the struggle for justice is the most basic as well as most critical. Despite all our progress and concomitant increases in life expectancy, survival remains precarious for many around the world. If current trends continue, 69 million children will die before their fifth birthdays between 2016 and 2030, with almost half of them in their first month itself. Even worse, 'for too many babies, their day of birth is also their day of death' (IGME 2015). Many who would be fortunate to survive until adulthood would not be able to have a 'fair innings' either, to use Alan Williams' (1997) phrase—77 per cent of deaths in the least developed countries happen before the age of 70 years vis-à-vis 29 per cent in more developed, with India being at 62 per cent (UNDP 2017, for the period 2015–20). 'In the long run we are all dead', as John Maynard Keynes once remarked. The question, however, for many of us is—until when will we survive, and under what circumstances?

The precariousness of survival is not as much about fate or destiny—or even lack of healthcare—as it is about deep-rooted inefficiencies and inequities that characterize our political, economic, social, cultural, and other arrangements. There have been substantial, systematic, and persistent inequities in the chances and conditions of survival between as well as within developing and developed countries and groups. However, there have been profound inefficiencies, too, that have adversely affected, in different measures, the chances of children from a diverse set of backgrounds to realize their optimal potentials. As a result, although survival is a much bigger issue for the disadvantaged groups, it also remains a concern in the case of the privileged as well, as we illustrate further. Survival and lack of opportunities to realize optimal potentials are key issues facing a vast majority of people, particularly in the developing world—it should, therefore, be a central concern of justice as well. In fact, as we argue in this book, they are prime instances of injustice and neglect of justice on the part of governments in developing countries in particular. Shots of vaccinations will not be enough—children deserve a shot of justice to survive, lead reasonably long, healthy, and productive lives and be able to realize their optimal potential, an opportunity every child in the world deserves.

It is a matter of great shame that we still have to worry about saving children in their first few days and years of life. The international development community has facilitated dramatic reductions in child mortality over the decades, especially through the Millennium Development Goals (MDGs). However, partly due to the continued challenge of child mortality, it has not been able to go beyond bare survival and flag issues related to children's quality of life and holistic development. Also, it has, wittingly or unwittingly, promoted a biomedical and technocratic approach to child mortality and underplayed fundamental inequities of human survival. It is not simply about bringing children to the brink of survival beyond the age of five and breathing a sigh of relief at having achieved our targets (under MDG 4 or Sustainable Development Goal 3 [SDG 3], for instance). What about the quality of survival, the persistent vulnerabilities of survival beyond the age of five years, and missed opportunities for addressing the enormous intergenerational inequalities that childhood offers?

If public action is able to ensure a certain level of equal treatment for all children, the economic or educational background of households—critical indicators of child survival in developing societies particularly—would matter much less and get children off to a much less unequal start. The literature on early child development (ECD) has demonstrated the impact of early achievement on adult life—'many children raised in disadvantaged environments start behind and stay behind' (Heckman and Kautz 2013). What are we doing to reduce the massive inequalities in such early achievement? What about the unrealized optimal potential of billions of survivors, not to talk of millions whose potential is buried with them prematurely? Bare survival cannot be the end of policy. A paradigm shift in development policy and practice is needed if it has to match with the aspirations of people. The predominant development policy and practice has failed to help developing countries reap their demographic dividends due to its short-sightedness and has led to a widespread sense of being left behind, given significant and persistent inequities in early achievement; to betrayed aspirations of social mobility of millions who try to compensate for their shortcomings in early achievement.

The long-standing problem of child mortality—and profound inequities in the span and quality of survival—cannot be fundamentally addressed with short-sighted policies and short-term measures. We have to take every human life seriously. We cannot have one set of development standards for children of privileged, and another for those of underprivileged, backgrounds. Children around the world deserve to be viewed and treated equally—every child should have the opportunity to realize their optimal potential. 'Human flourishing', as Aristotle argued, 'is the end of all political activity'. Public policy should not stop at anything short of that. The prevention of child mortality is the first step in the pursuit of justice; public policy has to aim at realization of optimal potentials of children even within the narrow ambit of a child survival policy. Its broader concern has to be with unequal chances as well as the conditions of survival so that we begin moving towards addressing the larger issue of intergenerational inequalities and fragility which threatens global development, peace, and stability. From a human perspective, children, rather than 'the basic structure of society', as Rawls argued, should be 'the primary subject of justice' (Rawls 1971: 3).

Why Is Child Mortality Unjust?

Neither popular nor academic discourses on justice have specifically considered child mortality as an instance of injustice, nor obviously have those dealing with it at national or international levels. Therefore, some justification of it is required, to begin with.

To start with, every preventable child death, irrespective of background, is unjust. Although there is a clear gradient in under-five child deaths and nutrition by socioeconomic status (Figure 1.1), deaths or

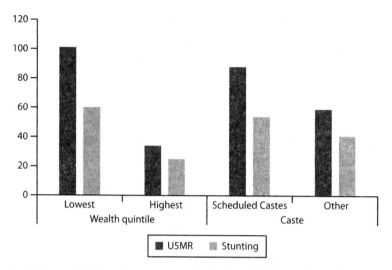

FIGURE 1.1   U5MR and Percentage of Under-Five Children Malnourished
(Stunted) by Selected Wealth Indices and Castes, India, NFHS-3 (2005–6)
Source: NFHS-3 national report.
Note: Stunting represents height-for-age below −2 SD (as defined by the
International Reference Population median).

stunting among under-five children from the highest wealth quintile or
the so-called upper caste ('other' in the caste category) background cannot be ignored just because their parents/guardians are privileged. As
we argued, children—not their parents—should be the primary subjects
of justice, particularly when we are dealing with justice for children.
'Every child has the inherent right to life', guaranteed in Article 6 of
the Convention on the Rights of the Child (CRC), which was adopted
by the United Nations in 1989 and is considered 'the most widely and
rapidly ratified human rights treaty in history'.[2] Furthermore, one
can argue that justice is *not just* about group/individual inequalities,
but also between an individual's actual status and his or her optimal
potential—what we might refer to as 'intra-individual inequality'. This
is the approach to justice that is argued for in this book. As part of
this approach, we also attempt to balance the concerns of equity and

[2] http://www.unicef.org/crc/index_30229.html (accessed 4 June 2012).

efficiency—inefficiency, as we argue later, tends to hurt the less privileged more than the privileged and is, thus, an indirect contributor to inter-group/individual disparities. Child mortality is not just a result of inequities, but also inefficiencies, and because it is a violation of 'the inherent right to life', it is unjust for all concerned. For an inclusive approach to justice—so that no one is left behind as far as the realization of optimal potentials is concerned—we need to take all types of groups and individuals into consideration. The backlash against the politics of social justice is due to the exclusion of the stereotypically privileged. Every preventable death—of a child or, for that matter, adult—is unjust and needs to be duly regarded in the public pursuit of justice.

From a philosophical perspective, preventable child mortality is unjust, whether one subscribes to equality of opportunity, that of outcomes, or of anything else between the two ends of the spectrum. We refer to these positions in some detail in the next section of this chapter, and discuss them in detail in the next chapter. The identification and redressal of injustice is premised on the notion of responsibility, a central theme in modern theories of justice. A particular process or outcome can be termed unjust only if some person or group of persons, beyond the concerned individual or group, can be held responsible 'for bringing it about or allowing it to come about' (Hayek 2013: 198). To the extent an individual is himself responsible, the question of justice does not arise since that person is regarded as responsible for his own state of affairs. However, as far as the particular instance of child mortality is concerned, there are basically two parties that can be held responsible—parents or guardians and the State. Even if under-five children die due to an action of their own, they cannot still be held responsible for their own death, even if none of the above two also can be held responsible. In such a case, it would simply be regarded as unfortunate, that is, occurring due to ill-fortune or luck, and beyond the capability of responsible parties to prevent it. Why children are not responsible has been discussed from a philosophical perspective towards the end of the chapter.

International declarations and conventions on the rights of children—from the Declaration of the Rights of the Child (1924) to the CRC—have held parents or guardians responsible for the 'special safeguards and care' that children need, with the state rendering appropriate assistance as required, 'in accordance with national conditions and within their means'. Even with respect to the right to life, as enshrined in the CRC, or the general right to life guaranteed in respective national constitutions of the top five contributors to under-five deaths in the world—India, China, Nigeria, Pakistan, and Bangladesh[3] (see Table 3.1 in Chapter 3)—the role of the State, either vis-à-vis addressing the shortfall in care and support that children need, or in monitoring and ensuring that children across the spectrum are able to enjoy an equal right to life, has remained ambiguous. China's constitution is the only exception in this case—it clearly makes protection of children the responsibility of the State, which it appears to have fulfilled well, reflected in a massive 89 per cent decline in the annual number of under-five deaths between 1990 and 2015 vis-à-vis 64 per cent in India (Table 3.1).

The right to life is the most fundamental constitutional entitlement of every citizen, and States are morally obliged—even if not legally, in a very strict sense—to make their best efforts to prevent premature mortality, especially at such early stages. States derive their moral sovereignty *primarily* from their ability to protect their citizens, not from protecting their borders. Ronald Dworkin, one of the most distinguished ethical and legal philosophers of the twentieth century, started out his *Sovereign Virtue* (2002: 1) with a categorical statement: 'No government is legitimate that does not show equal concern for the fate of all those citizens over whom it claims dominion and from whom it claims allegiance. Equal concern is the sovereign virtue of political community—without it government is only tyranny.' Even if the role of the State was limited to addressing the shortfall in parents' capability to save their children, most under-five deaths would still be the responsibility of the State as most parents would have done their best, as they deem fit, to keep their children alive. In addition, the

---

[3] 'No person shall be deprived of his life or personal liberty except according to procedure established by law' (India, Article 21). 'The State promotes the all-round development of children and young people, morally, intellectually and physically'; 'marriage, the family and mother and child are protected by the State' (China, Articles 46 and 49). 'Every person has a right to life' (Nigeria, Section 33). 'No person shall be deprived of life or liberty save in accordance with law' (Pakistan, Article 9). And, 'no person shall be deprived of life or personal liberty save in accordance with law' (Bangladesh, Article 32).

State is squarely responsible for the structural determinants of child survival (such as political and economic systems), which have a strong bearing on parental education, wealth, neighbourhood, and other intermediate determinants of child survival. If we follow this line of argument, the responsibility for child survival would eventually be that of the State. The family is 'the natural environment for the growth and well-being' of children (United Nations General Assembly 1989), but holding parents responsible for their children essentially 'rests on expediency rather than principle' (Friedman 1955).[4] By taking care of their children, parents not only ensure the continuation of their families, they also ensure 'the orderly production and reproduction of society' (Rawls 2008). Therefore, from the perspective of future demographic and development dynamics too, there is a strong case for the States to own responsibility for the future of their nation, their future human capital. The failure of the international system and development narrative to hold the States responsible—in unequivocal terms—is one of the fundamental causes for the persistent challenge of child survival and, to a degree, intergenerational inequalities.

States—and with them international organizations—have found it convenient to focus on immediate determinants and addressing them through cost-effective measures. In fact, discussions of justice are, in many cases, confined to inequality in access to healthcare. Children from poor backgrounds are seen as unable to access healthcare, while those from rich backgrounds are able to do so, hence the difference in outcomes. The proposal is that governments in developing countries should target their resources on those who cannot afford healthcare. This seems to address the immediate issue without having to get into the debate on why we have such inequality in children's backgrounds that inequality in access to healthcare comes about. Obviously, there is little to no discussion on the issue of quality healthcare, and the poor beneficiaries of government support are supposed to be thankful to the particular political party and government at the helm rather than

---

[4] Uneducated and poor parents tend to have more children, so high fertility is also a problem of national development. And, as per the demographic transition theory, it is only after declines in child mortality that declines in fertility usually happen. In other words, parents will generally have fewer children only when fewer of their children are dying.

question as to why they have to undergo the humiliation of government dole-outs and be satisfied with poor public provision of healthcare
(the humiliation of social justice).

Healthcare is not the only determinant of children's welfare or the
realization of optimal potentials. In fact, it plays a limited role. The
proper nutrition of a child and the mother at the immediate level
itself also has a central role to play in the child's health and development. There are public programs for that too. The Integrated Child
Development Services (ICDS) has been one of the flagship programmes
of the Government of India, and one of the largest in the world for
early child care and development. The quality of care in both public
health as well as ICDS centres in India is well documented and is not
part of this discussion. However, two questions need to be raised:
Why should poor children be entitled to poor quality healthcare and
nutrition and be unable to come out of the trap of intergenerational
poverty and inequality (those whose parents can afford get world-class
healthcare and education within India itself, widening the inequalities)?
What is the government doing to address non-income determinants (for
example, widespread discrimination that women, the so-called lower
castes, tribes, minorities, and others face and which negatively affects
their opportunities and outcomes, preventing them from realizing their
optimal potentials)? Resources for the poor are not the only support
that one would expect from governments—curbing discrimination is, at
times, a much bigger issue which they need to tackle to enable children
and adults realize their optimal potentials.

So, even within the limited sphere of healthcare, we would have
to deal with the intermediate and structural determinants as well as
the economic, political and social inequities and discriminations that
characterize them, if we are to consider issues of inequality in access
to quality care. The same applies to the issue of basic nutrition as well.
If parents are victims of injustice, so are their children—and so are the
chances and conditions of their survival. Even the otherwise privileged
parents would be victims of injustice when they lack the capability to
prevent the death of their children—whom most of them would do
anything in their capacity to save as well as to provide the best of life
and opportunities that they can maximally afford. Every preventable
child death is unjust, and the State is supposed to assume and act on its
responsibility to try its best to save each and every citizen.

Significance of Theories of Justice

We have some excellent book-length works that have analysed implications of the various theories of justice for the meaning and pursuit of health, health rights, the design of health policy,[5] and some recent work applying Sen's capability approach for the particular case of children.[6] However, this is the first book that invokes modern theories of justice in the context of 'ironic' inequalities in child survival from a developing country perspective, poses a challenge to several dominant notions of equality and justice, and tries to understand the policy implications of grounding these theories. More broadly, it calls for several justifications concerning the engagement of theories of justice, especially when the issue is urgent and there seems little time and scope for philosophizing on it. While providing these justifications, this section also highlights the significance of justice for child survival as well as need for well-reasoned theories—and not just a sense—of justice to decide what justice means, generally and specifically, for child survival. We will do this by raising and responding to some of the major objections that one could raise broadly on the engagement of notions of justice and particularly on normative theories of justice, in the context of child survival.

1. Biomedical, cost-effective interventions, and managerial solutions (for example, governance and efficiency of healthcare systems) can help us in saving millions of lives, as some researchers, state agencies, and non-governmental organizations portray them to be.[7] So there is no need for the theories of justice.

---

[5] Some prominent examples are Daniels (1985, 2008); Daniels, Kennedy, and Kawachi (1999); Faden and Powers (2008); Ruger (2009); Venkatapuram (2011).

[6] For instance, see Biggeri, Ballet, and Comim (2011); Bojer 2000; Graf, MacMullen, and Schweiger (2015); Hart, Biggeri, and Babic (2015); Leßmann, Otto, and Ziegler (2011); Macleod (2010), some of the major books on children from a capability perspective.

[7] This is how the issue of child mortality is largely viewed in India. For instance, Ramani et al. (2010) argue that if 'certain managerial issues' are addressed, we can 'satisfactorily' reduce child mortality and morbidity in the country.

2. Many of us, across ideological persuasions, could agree that preventable deaths of children are morally wrong and intolerable, and we should do all we can to save their lives. Where is the need to invoke theories of justice?

3. Our sense of justice clearly tells us that such deaths are unjust due to the fact that most of them are systematic, consistent, and preventable, and hence there is no requirement to dwell on the theories of justice.

4. Child survival is a result of socioeconomic development and social justice, which are pursued outside the health sector— why bring this discussion in the context of a child survival policy?

5. Despite socioeconomic disparities in child mortality, the crisis appears to be widespread, at least in regions such as north India (where majority of the deaths are taking place). This is considering that it is quite high even among male, rich, upper caste, urban, Hindu populations, who are relatively better off than their respective counterparts, at a general level, if not in every case. Where do theories of justice fit into this?

6. Theories of justice, by and large, do not treat children as concerns of justice, and hence child survival does not fall within their purview.

Let us deal with these potential objections, all of which are quite valid in their own right, given the dominant narrative on child mortality and survival.

For many international organizations working on child survival in India and elsewhere, most prominently the Bill and Melinda Gates Foundation (BMGF), vaccinations hold the key. Discussions on health and child survival in India are predominantly of a techno-managerial nature and convey an impression that there is little relevance of going into the structural, or even intermediate, causes of child mortality. The official Indian medical establishment opposes any move to even let social scientists have any prominent role on health issues (response of a prominent Indian demographer), although in official documents like ICMR (2007), it displays a concern with multidisciplinarity in health research.

Determinants of Child Survival

When child mortality acquires the stature of a crisis, as in the case of South Asia and sub-Saharan Africa, the biological and medical causes of death are symptomatic of problems not only with the finances of a particular state, but with its structure, institutions, values, and processes at a more fundamental level, as well as with that of the global system in a limited way.[8] In a crisis, it is wise to undertake interventions that can contain the crisis, but it is also wise not to stop at them and go beyond to identify and address the root causes. Healthcare and healthcare systems offer critical remedial measures to address the immediate biological determinants of child survival, but intermediate and structural determinants are beyond their scope. One could also make a case here in favour of prevention beyond cure. In fact, justice is a concern even at the level of addressing the immediate determinants—for instance, do we ignore vulnerable children belonging to highest wealth quintile or upper castes (refer to Figure 1.1)? If ability to afford healthcare is regarded as the central premise based on which the State assumes responsibility on the issue of child survival, how do we tackle deaths of children happening among economically or socially privileged but uneducated parents (parental education being a critical determinant of child survival)? This

[8] Cuba (6) had a lower under-five mortality rate than the US (8) in 2010 (IGME 2011), despite long-standing sanctions on the former imposed by the latter, which shows that with political will at the national level, countries could achieve good health status, even if the global political or financial system is not very conducive for this purpose. Health researchers concerned with political economy explanations (for instance, Navarro and Shi 2001) as well as the socialists present Cuba, China, and the erstwhile USSR as examples of how health can flourish under social democratic/socialist systems. However, there are counter-examples too—for instance, in the Indian state of West Bengal, which had a communist government for more than three decades (1977–2011), health indicators were mediocre at best, while in Kerala, where power alternated between communists and the centrist Congress party, health indicators have been the best. There are obviously other structural factors at play along with political economy—for instance, geographical predispositions to health and illness, or cultural practices, as we discuss later in the case of tribals and Muslims in India—most importantly, political will, quite often brought about by strong public awareness and demand for better health.

is a very fundamental issue in India—it is not difficult to see poor health-care practices or lack of sanitation (other major determinants of child survival and health) among people of a rich or upper caste background in the rural areas, for instance. This also leads us to the issue of informed choice, which is central to responsibility and justice, and which unedu-cated parents are unable to make in the context of poor educational attainment and weak regulatory structures and implementational issues as far as medicines and food, for example, are concerned. Linked to this issue is the availability of safe alternatives to choose from. Modern allo-pathic healthcare system is one set of 'means' to child survival. There are other 'means'—the alternative systems of medicine—and there is no reason why we should simply discredit and discard them just because we have the former—which itself has been seen by some as a 'murder-ous absurdity' (Shaw 1909), 'a major threat to health' (Illich 1976), or a limited actor vis-à-vis other factors in the 'prevention of death and increase in expectation of life in the past three centuries' (McKeown 1979). We do not necessarily have to agree with these assessments of modern healthcare, but most of us will agree on the need to expand safe healthcare choices. The Government of India is taking steps to develop alternative systems of medicine on scientific bases by promoting clini-cal trials and better regulatory systems for them. Furthermore, studies have highlighted the 'prominent' role of non-biological, socioeconomic determinants even within the first week and month of life, as we discuss in Chapter 4. This is especially relevant in a context where healthcare is not universally provisioned, or easily and cheaply available, and access to most basic immediate determinants is also determined by people's socioeconomic characteristics. To address the persistent problem and patterns of child mortality, as they exist in countries like India, we need to have policies which are based on sound principles rather than unfounded whims and fancies of politicians and policymakers, as a result of which we address some issues and include some groups—and ignore others—arbitrarily.

Is a Blank Cheque Sufficient for Survival?

Again, the claim of doing whatever is required cannot be a whimsi-cal one and is in need of several primary justifications. For instance, what is the appropriate role of the State in this regard? What do we owe to it and what does it owe to us? By what principles should it allocate resources in the background of competing demands from various sectors of the economy or segments of the society as well as within the health sector? Child mortality is not the only challenge that health systems or the State in general have to address. The issue of distributional justice has its own set of questions to be addressed—for instance, (*a*) what level and nature of taxation is fair to raise adequate resources for child survival?; and (*b*) by what principle should the State distribute resources among deserving beneficiaries, as not everyone would be equally deserving? Theories of justice can help address several of these questions and enable sound and principled policymaking, as will be demonstrated in this volume. If we were concerned with government employees and their dependents in India, and the only thing that mattered were resources, the solution would not have been that difficult. While per capita public health expenditure reached INR 913 (around USD 14) during the financial year 2013–14 (MoHFW 2016), central government employees have been making government sign blank cheques for their healthcare and that of their dependents since the establishment of the Central Government Health Scheme (CGHS) in 1954. As for the poor, this is what an official of the Health and Family Welfare Department of India's largest and most populous state, Uttar Pradesh (UP), had to say—'They keep producing children and expect us to fill their stomachs'. This is despite the fact that it is due to social injustices, because people are poor, illiterate and experience high child mortality that they have more children. In 2017, in UP, India's biggest contributor to child deaths as well as the epicentre of numerous forms of social injustices, more than 100 children died in one hospital in a matter of few days in the chief minister's own district—oxygen supplies were discontinued due to long-pending payments. Talking of a blank cheque for survival in the context of such governmental attitudes is a mirage. It is precisely due to the structurally anti-poor policies that there are such gross inequities in the country in the first place. Otherwise, is it scarcity of resources which is preventing one of the top ten economies in the world—and the aspirant to be among the top three in the next 25 years[9]—that India is from according top priority to child survival

[9] India's Union Finance Minister Arun Jaitley's statement at an India–ASEAN meeting in New Delhi on 22 January 2018.

and flourishing? India is the only country among the top ten economies whose public expenditure on healthcare is lower than its military expenditure, as a percentage of GDP. China, despite being the world's second largest military spender after the US,[10] spends more on health. India's is a serious case of misplaced priority-setting and resource allocation—instead of correcting it, the Government of India actually cut down on the central health budget some time back, and is presenting and promoting a cost-effective intervention such as vaccination as the ultimate life-saving solution (Nadda 2015).

Policy advocates struggle for arguments to convince it to accord higher priority to health in general. Theories of justice can help us clearly determine the responsibilities of the State toward its citizens, and support policy advocacy on a much more fundamentally sound footing.

Sense or Theory of Justice?

Certainly, there can be little doubt that a systematic and consistent pattern of deaths among certain social groups, especially those that are preventable, makes it clear that social injustice is at work and we do not need much theorization to reach such a conclusion. However, things are not always that clear. Consider the following cases of child survival from the Indian context:

1. Despite large-scale displacement and discrimination that the Scheduled Tribes (STs) have faced, they were doing much better than the Scheduled Castes (SCs) or Dalits as well as the non-SCs and non-STs in rural Bihar in terms of infant mortality rate (IMR)—74, 120, and 88 respectively in 1978 and 78, 99, and 98 in 1984 (RGI 1983, 1989).
2. In West Bengal,[11] SCs (47) were doing much better in terms of their under-five mortality rate (U5MR) vis-à-vis the upper castes (UCs) (70).

---

[10] Constant 2011 USD (Stockholm International Peace Research Institute/SIPRI).

[11] All values in points 2 and 3 are from the third round of the National Family Health Survey (NFHS-3), 2005–6.

3. Infant mortality rate in a highly patriarchal state such as Haryana was better among females (43) than males (45), and in a relatively better state (in terms of the position of women) such as Tamil Nadu, it was almost the same for females and males (37.8 and 37.6 respectively). Females have a better chance at survival, so their mortality should ideally be lower; equal mortality rates signify discrimination against them. This has implications for the selection of an appropriate central focal variable, which we will discuss later.

4. Muslims have had an advantage in child survival despite the fact that they have been discriminated at various levels and have much worse access to modern healthcare and education. A number of explanations have been put forth for this—higher urbanization (Kulkarni 2010); taller stature, non-vegetarian diet, lesser likelihood of employment among Muslim mothers, higher treatment-seeking behaviour during diarrhoea, and lesser son-preference vis-à-vis Hindus (Bhalotra, Valente, and van Soest 2010); much less likelihood of open defecation among Muslims vis-à-vis Hindus (Geruso and Spears 2014). Geruso and Spears have argued that 'this one difference in sanitation can fully account for the large child mortality gap between Hindus and Muslims', much more than even the wealth effects. However, almost all these factors have more to do with internal community characteristics rather than public interventions.

Several questions can be raised vis-à-vis these cases: What are the policy implications of ST or Muslim advantage in child survival? Do their children deserve lesser policy attention and public resources because they have better survival chances (not due to public intervention, rather despite them)? Alternatively, should we rather discuss issues of justice vis-à-vis access to the determinants of child survival (equality of opportunity)? When access to the determinants of health is unjust, are outcomes also unjust, even if they are better off than that of those who are better off in terms of access to determinants? Should the primary focus of a child survival policy be on fair provision of determinants of health, health outcomes, or on something else? How do we design a just policy of child survival in the light of these cases? No principled policymaking for such cases is possible based on our sense of justice, while discussions in political philosophy, as demonstrated later, can prove to be quite helpful.

Given the disillusionment with justice, highlighted at the beginning of this chapter, and the strength of emotions with which both claims and counter-claims of justice are made, it is imperative to deal with the issue of *sense* of justice and injustice in greater detail. Let us ask: How far can our sense of justice take us? To what extent is it reliable? We, broadly, have two schools of thought on this.

The first school of thought relates to one of the most ardent proponents for sense of injustice in the twentieth century. For American legal philosopher, Edmond Cahn, although our sense of injustice is, like any other human capacity, 'finite and fallible', it is not just based on empathy and emotion. 'It simultaneously summons perception, reasoning, intelligence, and judgment—all the capacities that make for understanding and the application of sense' (Cahn 1966: 13–14). Likewise, the empathetic as well as the rational dimension of a sense of justice has been invoked, where 'sense' is equated with sentiment (*Rechtsgefühl*), as against sensation or mere feeling (*Rechtsempfindung*), and so is not necessarily irrational (Dubber 2006). Way back in 1762, Rousseau, in his *Émile*, perceived the sense of justice as 'a true sentiment of the heart enlightened by reason' (Rawls 1963: 281). From this perspective, it is important to appreciate that a 'sense', in this context, cannot be pitted against reason, as something essentially illusory, subjective, and senseless. Even further, while others have attributed an element of rationality to the sense of (in)justice, Cahn seems to support it as a sufficient guide in itself. And as far as our collective sense of (in)justice is concerned, we can also count Michael Walzer in this school of thought, inasmuch as he argues for a socially or culturally constructed conventional notion of (in)justice.[12] From his perspective, the Indian caste system would only be unjust if the Dalits, for instance, themselves see it in this way (Walzer 1983). If child mortality is not considered unjust by the citizens of India—which it is largely not—it would not be regarded so from this perspective.

---

[12] 'Every substantive account of distributive justice is a local account.... Since there is no way to rank and order these (meaningful) worlds (of various cultures) with regard to their understanding of social goods, we do justice to actual men and women by respecting their particular creations' (Walzer 1983: 314).

The second school of thought comprises those who, at a very broad level, believe that we do need a theory of (in)justice. However, as one would expect, there are several variations within this broad position. While none of the major political and legal philosophers seems to have argued for completely ignoring the sense of (in)justice in favour of a theory of justice, there are differing levels of emphases. Judith Shklar, for instance, has made a very strong case for giving the victim's sense of injustice its due. However, because 'victimhood has an irreducibly subjective component', she argues in favour of 'a full theory of injustice' (Shklar 1990: 36–8). At the other end of this spectrum is Ronald Dworkin, who, while arguing for generality, particularly against Walzer, maintains that 'we cannot leave justice to convention and anecdote' (Dworkin 1985: 220).[13] There are other positions in between these two. For instance, according to Sen, 'our sense of injustice could serve as a signal that moves us, but a signal does demand critical examination' (Sen 2009: viii). It seems that Sen takes a rudimentary view of the sense of injustice, as more of a moral feeling, which stands in need of clear articulation and rational scrutiny, and, therefore, of a theory of justice. Way back in 1861, Mill felt likewise, arguing that 'the feeling of justice might be a peculiar instinct, and might yet require, like our other instincts, to be controlled and enlightened by a higher reason' (Mill 1998). However, Rawls seems to end the dichotomy between a sense of (in)justice and a theory of justice by arguing that the former is shaped by the latter,[14] and may, therefore, help us identify (in)justice, although not in an absolute or objective sense.

While I do not share the scepticism of Mill, Dworkin, or Sen towards the sense of (in)justice, I also do not share the extreme optimism of Cahn, and think that we do need an objective criterion, which is out

---

[13] For him, 'political theory can make no contribution to how we govern ourselves except by struggling, against all the impulses that drag us back into our own culture, toward generality and some reflective basis for deciding which of our traditional distinctions and discriminations are genuine and which spurious, which contribute to the flourishing of the ideals we want, after reflection, to embrace, and which serve only to protect us from the personal costs of that demanding process' (Dworkin 1985: 219–20).

[14] In the Rawlsian perspective, 'a sense of justice is the capacity to understand, to apply, and to act from the public conception of justice which characterizes the fair terms of social cooperation' (Rawls 1985: 233).

there as a shared reference, for a reasoned identification of injustices and a clear articulation of justice. One can put forth several arguments in support of this standpoint. A few of these are discussed further.

The Problem of Perception

The sense of injustice needs a spark of perception that an injustice is being done. However, it is possible that many of us are not able to perceive injustice as a phenomenon in the first place, due either to low analytical skills or the complex and abstract nature and dimensions of injustice.[15] It is also possible that based on our values and indoctrination, we do perceive the phenomenon, but do not normatively interpret it as injustice. Although it may be wrong to believe that even in its heyday, all low-caste members simply acquiesced in their exploitation by members of the upper castes—as some functionalists would have us believe—many of them did, and a few possibly continue to, accept it as their fate or misfortune, but not injustice. Another possibility is that injustices, especially those with a religious sanction, have been committed without much resentment for such a long period of time, and in such a widespread manner, that they take the shape of a tradition, and both perpetrators and victims come to see them as normal and fine, rather than unjust. At the same time, it is also possible that, due to a long history of injustice, as on the basis of caste, victims might develop a heightened sense of injustice after some empowerment and view injustice even in cases where it may just not exist.[16] The problem of objective and subjective perception can also be invoked in the case of victimizers, though this is more debatable, since victimizers, being in a leading position, can couch their actions in a language of justice.

[15] It needs to be highlighted here that sociologists as well as other social scientists have worked extensively on issues related to social stratification, exclusion, discrimination, inequality, and so on, which could be used as the empirical basis for the normative identification of injustices. However, these insights have largely been neglected by moral and political philosophers, including Sen, despite arguing for a focus on actual lives that people are able to lead.

[16] A prominent Dalit leader in India once told me that he was discriminated at the New York airport because he was a Dalit. When I asked him how this was possible, he said that the upper castes have also influenced the Americans now!

Under such situations, we cannot simply counter the language or the purported sense of justice with our sense of injustice, at an institutional level, though we can surely, and maybe more effectively, do that by coming out on the streets, through the ballot or other such indirect means. Formally, we need an objective criteria to tell us not only *what* is unjust, but *how* and *why*, in a systematic way, especially when injustice is complex and abstract. Although child deaths are patterned and preventable, they are not seen as unjust in India. On the other hand, a major rail accident, involving the death of a few people, leads to public outcry and demands for the resignation of the railway minister. We have never asked for the resignation of a health minister despite under-five child deaths in millions, year after year, for several decades. This is probably one of the major reasons why such deaths have continued in this manner.

The Problem of Empowerment

As Shklar (1990) herself admits, there might be cases in which the victims of injustice are *unwilling* to identify themselves as such, either due to fear of the victimizers, helplessness in the face of injustice, to maintain a positive perspective of themselves or of life in general,[17] because of cultural or religious considerations, and so on. Social and political psychologists have conducted studies to understand reactions—and their context—of the victims to injustice. For instance, Moore (1978) discussed the sociological, psychological, and historical factors that could explain the presence or absence of a sense of injustice or 'moral outrage' among people at, or near, the bottom of a social order. Morton Deutsch, who worked on the social psychology of justice for nearly half a century, co-authored a paper on victims' and victimizers' differential sensitivity to injustice and the conditions required for 'awakening the sense of injustice' among them in an unjust relationship (Deutsch and Steil 1988). We often find champions of justice, usually from civil society, stand up in favour of victims, but that depends on how these champions of justice view justice or injustice, and there is rarely any discussion between them and on whose behalf they stand up on this

---

[17] 'Many of us would rather reorder reality than admit that we are the helpless objects of injustice' (Shklar 1990: 38).

issue. The issue of empowerment is relevant even in this benevolent relationship.

The Problem of Vested Interests

Unlike the state of nature in the traditional 'social contract', or the hypothetical world of Rawls's 'original position' (Rawls 2001: 11), our perceptions and sense of (in)justice in the actual world are neither shaped behind a 'veil of ignorance' of our natural possessions and social positions, nor always a perfect blend of reason and emotion in a Cahnian sense. Due to respective vested interests, it is possible that victims overplay their injustice or settle other scores in the name of injustice, while victimizers either underplay or completely dismiss it. We, therefore, need objective criteria in reference to which we can decide what is unjust, irrespective of the respective interests or positions of the parties involved.[18]

Having raised doubts regarding exclusive reliance on the sense of (in)justice, I would also like to mention that while theories of justice can bring clarity to policy and public debates on justice, it is eventually the citizens' sense and commitment to justice—based on well-reasoned arguments and theories of justice—that is going to ensure justice in policy and public life. Theories of justice, on their own, cannot bring about justice or reduce injustices in the world. Therefore, in a way, there is not really a dichotomy between sense and theories of justice— they have their complementary roles to play in the pursuit of justice. However, politicization of social justice based on vested interests is something that citizens of all backgrounds need to be particularly

---

[18] The institutions and processes of legal justice have often come to the rescue of victims of social injustice, but in my view, social justice is a much broader concept and concern than legal justice. To use the emerging international language on health, social justice is about 'whole-of-society' and 'whole-of-government' approach. As a loud suggestion, national constitutions should be imbued with well-argued and reasoned principles of justice since they serve as common reference documents for governments, judiciary and citizens alike. In addition, to an extent, they already are. The debate on social justice, like social justice itself, should be made more and more inclusive to be more objective and legitimate.

careful about—politicians have used it for vote-bank politics, sowing seeds of social discord by pitting one or more group against others. Even those politicians who counter-mobilize these 'others' against the politics of social justice are equally involved in its politicization and resultant social conflict.

General Versus Specific Justice and Development

A broader pursuit of social justice or socioeconomic development would enhance chances of child survival. There is ample evidence for it, and is part of the structural determinants of child survival. However, there are several points to be noted here. One, what do we mean by social justice when we say that it is pursued in a broader sphere, beyond the sphere of health? If we go by the capability perspective to justice, then health capabilities are an integral part of the program of social justice, while capability to avoid premature mortality is foremost in that framework. Health does not only allow us to be productive citizens, it is valuable in itself.

Similarly, child mortality is not important because it contributes to reduced fertility—as Indian policymakers have seen it—but because it is an end in itself. An important justification for the State is protection and promotion of human life. Two, even if we have a narrow resourcist view of social justice, still, the struggle for social justice has to be waged in various spheres, with child survival being the most fundamental of them (social justice would not mean much unless we are alive). Furthermore, to an extent, the pursuit of justice rests on peculiar demands of various spheres. With reference to child survival, justice would also involve provision of those determinants, like child and maternal healthcare, which would not be part of pursuit of justice in the sphere of employment, for example. As far as socioeconomic development is concerned, it is not necessary that it works equally to the benefit of all sections of the society. Again, sector-specific interventions are needed in addition to the general ones. We cannot confine our analysis to broad institutional arrangements which are supposed to improve the chances of child survival, and have to deal with it in its own right, as an issue of priority and not as one of subsidiary consequence. Forget the politics of social justice, even theories of justice have not given children their due, as we discuss in some detail in the next few sections.

Justice in Crisis

The relevance of an appropriate theory of justice cannot be more than with reference to this issue. Who should we help out in the sphere of child survival? Should we only help the poor? If equal concern for the fate of all citizens is what Dworkin (2002) refers to as the *sovereign virtue* of the political community, we need to ask ourselves here: what does an equal concern in the sphere of child survival mean? These questions demand explicit ethical analysis and a strong basis of justification for an equitable and efficient allocation of available public resources. They also highlight the fact that deprivation is context-specific, and not always universal, and therefore a reliance on universal measures of deprivations could have negative effects within certain contexts like the one we are concerned with here. For instance, so-called upper castes in India have an advantage over lower castes in many spheres, but this does not mean that they would also have an advantage over them in the sphere of child survival in every context. This is by no means an irrelevant issue in the Indian context particularly where serious reservations have been raised about the affirmative action/reservation system prevalent in the country. Generally, the conceptual bases and identification of deserving beneficiaries in India has been an issue of great controversy. At the same time, we need to keep in mind that socioeconomic differentials in exposure to risks and outcomes exist even in poor-performing countries and states, and we need to decide what needs to be equalized. Theories of justice would not perhaps be more relevant elsewhere—the crisis, in itself, in large part, is an outcome of injustice and some serious structural reforms designed to address issues of both efficiency and equity need to be put in place. The scene from the Hollywood movie, *I, Robot* (2004), in which the robot rescues the protagonist, a Detective Del Spooner, from water after a car accident and lets the little girl drown because her chances of survival were lower than the former, illustrates how issues of justice are important even in acute situations of crisis. For the realization of MDG 4, some countries were accused of adopting a 'low-hanging fruit' approach, given their inclination to prioritize focus on those who could help them achieve the national target of child mortality quickly. Decisions based on justice and equity require careful consideration, otherwise one could end up adding to rather than reducing injustice. Obviously, one is not expected to think about theories of justice in such acute situations as above. However, if our sense of justice is guided by well-reasoned principles of justice, instant decisions too are likely to be more reasonably just rather than random and impulsive.

Crisis of Justice

Having argued so far about the relevance of theories of justice, let me also discuss why mainstream Western theories of justice have remained largely irrelevant in the context of real-life injustices as well as for the particular case of children. Amartya Sen's approach to justice is an exception, even if a limited one, and we highlight in the final section of this chapter why, therefore, we have chosen to focus on it.

Neglect of the Real World

Political philosophers like Rawls were profoundly concerned with the removal of 'great evils of human history' and the 'gravest forms of political injustice' (Rawls 2008). The problem, however, is that political philosophers have rarely tried to understand the dynamics and processes of the real world, of the complex ways in which various agents view justice or injustice, and operate to produce and perpetuate them, or identify actual conditions that would be necessary for enhancements of justice, or the implications that their theories might have for various sets of people in a given context. While Sen has argued for taking the empirical fact of pervasive human diversity (of internal characteristics as well as external circumstances) into consideration while deciding on a central focal variable of justice (Sen 1995), he has largely remained confined to philosophical–empirical facts without going ahead to consider anthropological–empirical facts too in discussions of justice.

While political philosophers developed their own theories of justice, they cared little—and in several cases, not at all—about what ordinary people, policymakers or others think of justice. Even if they would not prefer to go 'out into broad and open land'—as the restless Faust in his chair and by his desk wished—a vast body of literature exists on ordinary people's sense, perceptions, judgements, experiences of, and reactions to, what they perceive as (in)justice, produced by social and political psychologists, notably since the 1960s (Mikula 1984).[19] What are the 'social and historical conditions under which moral outrage' does and does not appear (Moore 1978)? How do people think of justice without the Rawlsian 'veil of ignorance', of their particular positions and interests? Such issues would have a bearing not only on the operationalization of a particular theory of justice, but also on its conceptualization, content, and consequences too (Miller 1991). Empirical studies of justice can, as Elster (1995) argued, influence the structure of the scaffolding that professional theorists of justice construct during the process of elaboration, and shape the focus of their arguments too. Public reasoning has been given an important place in these theories, but people are expected to reason within the broad framework proposed by them. What about public reasoning on what constitutes justice itself?

According to Jürgen Habermas (1996: 43), the German critical theorist and an outstanding philosopher and social scientist of our time, theories of justice have lost 'touch with the reality of contemporary societies and thus have difficulties in identifying the conditions necessary for the realization of these principles'. The problem is not just about the realization of principles of justice in the real world—it is about their very conceptualization in the first place. 'When a theory of justice takes a directly normative approach and attempts to justify the principles of a well-ordered society by operating beyond existing institutions and traditions, it faces the problem of how its abstract idea of justice can be brought into contact with reality' (Habermas 1996: 197–8). Rawls's theory is 'an example of the complementary difficulties

---

[19] One such exploratory study was carried out in 1991 under the International Social Justice Project at Humboldt-Universität zu Berlin by social scientists from Russia, Poland, Hungary, Bulgaria, Estonia, Slovenia, Czechoslovakia, Germany, Great Britain, Netherlands, United States, and Japan, who studied popular beliefs and attitudes to social, economic and political justice in their countries by means of large-scale opinion surveys. An excellent example of an empirical–analytical social psychological study on 'what people regard as unjust' is Mikula, Petri, and Tanzer (1990) and Lipkus (1992). For a brief history of justice research and relevant social psychological perspectives, refer to Kazemi and Törnblom (2008) and Deutsch (1983). One could also refer to the journal, *Social Justice Research*, for relevant studies. In the Indian context, recently, the Calcutta Research Group published a four-volume study on governmental and popular notions of social justice (Samaddar 2009).

that confront a philosophical discourse of justice carried out in a purely normative fashion' (Habermas 1996: 43), the '*prescriptivism* of a rational law whose normative arguments disregarded historical particularity and sociocultural facts' (p. 44; emphasis as per original), and was eventually faced with the 'impotence of the ought' (p. 56). 'At stake is the old problem of how the rational project of a just society', which is developed 'in abstract contrast to an obtuse reality', develops 'bridges between the two universes of discourse' (p. 57), the normative and the empirical. This reminds me of a classical Bollywood song from the 1957 movie, *Dekh Kabira Roya*—'*Humse aaya na gaya, tumse bulaya na gaya, fasla pyar mein dono se mitaya na gaya*' ('I could not come, you could not invite, both of us could not remove the distance in love'). Despite the inspiration from and motivational concern with the real world of injustices, there has been a severe divide between the theories of justice and the world of actual injustices.

Neglect of Injustice

Related to this perhaps is also the conceptual neglect of the notion of injustice and focus on utopian notions of justice. More than two and a half thousand years ago, Plato asked the question, 'what is justice', and initiated political philosophy in the Western world (Barry 1989). However, rarely since has a similar question been asked about 'injustice'[20] and most political philosophers have gone on to take a negative view of it, as the absence of justice (Wolgast 1987). If the basic structure and institutions of the society become just, so seems to be their argument, there will be no or little room left for injustice—social or behavioural. Even in his 'realistic Utopia', Rawls insisted that 'once political injustice has been eliminated by following just (or at least decent) social policies and establishing just (or at least decent) basic institutions, these great

---

[20] Shklar (1990: 21–4) argues that 'any effort to think about injustice in all its magnitude must begin with Plato', and 'his is the most radical of all rejections of the normal model [which largely confines itself to discussions of justice]'. Injustice, according to Plato (as cited in Shklar), 'is first and foremost a cognitive problem. Our inability to know the whole and to understand what a rational society would be in its entirety and in every one of its relations renders us incapable of establishing a just order.'

evils [unjust wars, oppression, religious persecution, slavery, etc.] will eventually disappear' (Rawls 2008). As a result, he and others in the social contract tradition have been preoccupied with the character-ization of perfectly just institutional arrangements, which according to them will also help us in the identification of unjust or 'imperfect societies',[21] and the extent to which they depart or deviate from 'perfect justice' without justifiable reasons (Rawls 1971). Inasmuch as political philosophy has not given 'injustice' its due (Shklar 1990; Simon 1995), it could be said to have progressed little, in this respect, since the time of Plato (Lötter 1993).

Unless we see injustice as mere absence or 'breakdown' of justice, theories of perfect justice, on their own, cannot tell us what is unjust (Shklar 1990). According to Sen, 'the diagnosis of injustice does not demand a unique identification of "the just society"', and that the question, 'what is a just society?', is neither a good starting point nor a plausible end point (Sen 2009). More importantly, even if we accord primacy to the idea of justice, the theory of a perfectly just society may, at best, tell us which societies, on the whole, are not perfectly just (though here too, the issue of the ranking of unjust societies would be quite problematic, and not straightforward, as assumed by proponents of perfect justice). They are incapable of offering us any guidance for identification of the diverse individual and social practices of injustices, especially when they are complex and subtle. They also cannot tell us what constitutes an act of injustice, or provide a criteria which can be used to distinguish calamity from injustice and vice versa, or situations in which calamity may take the shape of injustice, so on and so forth. With a focus on the basic structure of society and its institutions, the contractarian theories of justice have nothing to say about actual non-institutional practices, except for the assumption that they would fall in line once the basic structure is just. Ask any field-based sociologist or social scientist, well versed in issues of social stratification and exclu-sion, and he or she will easily tell you how naïve such an assumption is. One could also argue that, if 'it is perfectly possible, and arguably much easier, to identify particular, serious injustices than it is to articulate a theory of justice or even to have much idea of what a perfectly just

---

[21] Plato (2003) describes four types of 'imperfect societies'—Timarchy, Oligarchy, Democracy, and Tyranny—in Books VIII and IX of *Republic*.

society would look like' (Horton 2005: 31), there is even a stronger case for focusing our energies on injustices and making societies less unjust.

However, as legal philosophers have tried to be in touch with social reality (such as Habermas 1996), they and those concerned with actual injustices and deprivations have argued for the primacy of injustice, since without it, there would be no reason to think of justice in the first place. For some within this perspective,[22] justice *as an ideal* is 'a hopelessly ambiguous concept' (Cahn 1966: 11), and justice *as a process* is best seen negatively, as the absence of injustices.[23] This does not simply pertain to 'the grammar of justice', but has profound implications for the way we conceive of reducing injustices and enhancing justice in the world. The main focus shifts from the grand task of conceptualizing perfect justice to an earthly identification and removal of manifest and remediable injustices. The question to be asked is not how we could make, let us say, Indian society perfectly just, rather how it could it be made less unjust. The more injustices are removed, the more just the Indian society becomes (Sen 2009). Although in the context of the philosophy of law, Hayek (2013: 207–8) characterizes such a standpoint quite well:

> The fact that, though we have no positive criteria of justice, we do have negative criteria which shows us what is unjust, is very important in several respects. It means, in the first instance, that, though the striving to eliminate the unjust will not be a sufficient foundation for building up a wholly new system of law, it can be an adequate guide for developing an existing body of law with the aim of making it more just ... a negative test which enables us progressively to eliminate what is unjust.... [W]e can always only endeavour to approach truth, or justice, by persistently eliminating the false or unjust, but can never be sure that we have achieved final truth or justice.

There are many practical benefits of an injustice-oriented approach. First and foremost, it has the potential of promoting justice in the real

---

[22] These two positions have been broadly outlined here, but apart from their general focus on justice or injustice respectively, there are major differences among philosophers within each broad position.

[23] Wolgast (1987: 126–7) has also shown how justice cannot also be considered as an 'original state' or equilibrium, from which injustice is a digression, requiring readjustment of the scales of justice.

world (as against the hypothetical world of the social contract) by making us focus on actual injustices rather than on generic problems that justice is supposed to overcome. Second, the possibility of removing or reducing injustices is significantly higher than the creation of even a remotely perfect just society, and this has the potential to not only motivate us toward action, but toward improving the plight of those who suffer injustices here and now. Striving for an illusory goal like perfectly just society can lead us to disillusionment not just with a theory of justice, but generally with an aspiration for justice itself. Third, at least as far as manifest injustices are concerned, there is probably a higher chance of reaching an 'overlapping consensus' on injustice than 'a political conception of justice' (Rawls 1987). Such a consensus would provide us with a positive starting point, a common framework to engage with people from diverse groups and affiliations on potential solutions to such injustices. Fourth, even as justice is seen as 'something flat, without depth or dynamic vigour', 'a cold virtue', 'injustice is something we soon get steamed up about' (Lucas 1980: 4–5), and therefore possesses greater potential of motivating us to work towards making the world a less unjust place. Justice as an ideal, for Cahn (1949: 13), 'bakes no loaves', while a sense of injustice, even if imagined, produces warmth and movement in us.

Neglect of Children

Theories of justice have not given children their due. According to estimates provided by *World Population Prospects: The 2017 Revision* (UNPD 2017), there were 674 million children aged 0 to 4 years in the world in 2015—a little more than 9 per cent of world population. As per the provisional population totals from India's Census 2011, children aged 0 to 6 years constituted almost 159 million or 16 per cent of India's total population, of which nearly 83 million were males, 76 million females. If we go by the definition of the child provided by the CRC (every human being below the age of 18: article 1), we will have four times those numbers. How can we leave out such large parts of our populations from the purview of justice, especially when hundreds of millions of them continue to suffer the most abject forms of deprivations? The year 2006 was the first in human history in which less than 10 million children died before their fifth birthday. According to the International Labour

Organization's *Global Estimates of Child Labour* (ILO 2017), 152 million children aged 5–17 years in 2016 worked as child labourers—many as slaves, drug-traffickers, prostitutes, or child soldiers. The occurrence of child deprivation is not unique to developing nations, although it is most appalling there. In Organisation for Economic Co-operation and Development (OECD) countries, 13.5 per cent children (0–17 years) lived in income poverty, as per latest figures available in mid-2017, with that figure going over 20 per cent in the US (OECD Family Database), where highly sophisticated theories of justice have been developed and debated in recent decades. Neglect of children is part of the larger neglect of the concept as well as practice of injustice as well as the neglect of the real world. To envision a society 'well-ordered' as per the principles of justice, chosen behind an imaginary 'veil of ignorance', there has been an attempt to 'avoid needless complications' (Rawls 1971) of 'obtuse', 'resistant' (Habermas 1996), and 'messy' (Panini 2000) social realities and actual injustices, which carry the potential of producing a 'cynical' disenchantment with normative moorings.

International and national organizations long recognized that children need special protection and special rights, and their untiring efforts since the Universal Declaration of Human Rights in 1948 finally paved the way for the CRC in 1989, ratified by all countries, except US and Somalia. At the dawn of the new millennium, the United Nations General Assembly adopted the Millennium Declaration, calling for 'collective responsibility', in particular, towards 'the children of the world, to whom the future belongs'. However, most political philosophers have not seen children either as subjects of justice or as special cases for human rights. Since Rawls is widely seen as the greatest political philosopher of the twentieth century whose theory of justice led to widespread interest in issues of justice, his works are cited here as illustrative of the broader inclinations in the dominant modern political philosophical paradigm.

Rawls, like others, seems to have treated the issue of children with a degree of diffidence. For him, public policy and law in a democratic regime *should* support and regulate institutions that reproduce political society over time (including the family, arrangements for the rearing and education of children and general public health), children *should* enjoy inalienable 'basic rights' as 'future citizens', and parents *should* follow some 'conception' of justice or fairness in raising and treating them. However, the political 'principles' of justice do not apply to the internal life of the family, but to the basic structure of the society, of which family is a part. We have to, 'at some point', rely on the 'natural affection and goodwill of the mature family members' as far as children are concerned.[24] Though he explicitly talks about women's 'equal rights' as 'equal citizens', he does not in the case of children (Rawls 2008). Children have not been offered a better deal by other theorists of justice either, an issue that has been raised in other works on children and justice too.

To understand the neglect of children, we need to briefly touch upon discussions in political philosophy. In presenting a systematic critique of utilitarianism—the most prominent ethical theory of his time and for much of the modern period—and proposing an alternative theory of justice based on the traditional notion of the 'social contract', Rawls started out by raising the issue of the equalisandum—*what* is it that should be equalized across persons in a just society? This was posed later as 'equality of what?' by Amartya Sen in his 1979 Tanner Lecture on Human Values (Roemer 1996). In response to Rawls's 'social primary goods',[25] a number of metrics of justice were put forth, some of the influential ones being: Robert Nozick's libertarian 'rights' (1974), Sen's 'capabilities' (1979), Ronald Dworkin's 'bundle of resources' (1981), Richard Arneson's 'opportunity for welfare' (1989) and G.A. Cohen's 'midfare' (1993b).

There seem to be three major reasons for the exclusion of children from the scope of theories of justice. One, they have been concerned

---

[24] Okin (1989: 19) has powerfully argued that we cannot just 'rely on love, altruism, and generosity as the basis for family relations', making a case for 'just family structures as necessary for socializing children into citizenship in a just society'. Child psychologists and sociologists studying family and socialization would tell us how many of the gendered attitudes, for example, are engendered within the family since early childhood, which is equally true for children's attitudes towards race, caste, class, and so on.

[25] Social primary goods—or goods that 'every rational man is presumed to want', irrespective of his 'rational plan of life'—comprise 'rights and liberties, powers and opportunities, income and wealth' (Rawls 1971: 62), and the social 'bases of self-respect' (p. 303). Two aspects of Rawls's theory need to be highlighted here. One, his theory, like that of Dworkin as well as Nozick's,

with rational and responsible agents (Rawls 1971), those who are 'normal and fully cooperating members of society' (Rawls 1981, 1985, 1988, 1989), and children do not fit into this description (neither do a number of disabled and elderly people). Two, children, especially the smaller ones, are problematic for those theories of justice that focus on procedural fairness or advocate equal distribution of some resource(s), and hold citizens responsible for outcomes. In fact, according to Roemer (1996: 164), 'if one idea must be singled out as the most prominent in contemporary theories of distributive justice, it is that personal responsibility justifiably restricts the degree of outcome equality'. As far as children are concerned, they are not responsible agents and, therefore, outcome equality is difficult to restrict in their case. No preventable death of a child can be justified, no matter how fair the procedures and how equitable the distribution of any set of resources have been. Three, since modern theories of justice focus on individual justice, holding the interests of the individuals inviolable,[26] they cannot really argue that the fully cooperating members of society (parents) should sacrifice their personal liberties or resources for the sake of 'future citizens' (children) beyond a certain limit, although many of them do hold

---

is primarily means-, resource-, or opportunity-oriented, arguing in favour of 'pure procedural justice', which when followed, translates its fairness to outcomes, whatever they are. Two, for the notion of pure procedural justice to be applicable, 'it is necessary to set up and to administer impartially a just system of institutions' (Rawls 1971: 86–7) based on two principles of justice. According to the First Principle, 'each person is to have an equal right to the most extensive total system of equal basic liberties compatible with a similar system of liberty for all'. As per the Second Principle, 'social and economic inequalities are to be arranged so that they are both: (a) to the greatest benefit of the least advantaged, consistent with the just savings principle, and (b) attached to offices and positions open to all under conditions of fair equality of opportunity' (p. 302). The other important metric is Sen's, which is discussed at length in the following pages.

[26] Rawls started out his magnum opus by stating that 'each person possesses an inviolability founded on justice that even the welfare of society as a whole cannot override' (Rawls 1971: 3). Similarly, Nozick started out by asserting that 'individuals have rights, and there are things no person or group may do to them' (Nozick 1974: ix). Sen, too, focuses on 'individual advantage' (for example, Sen 1995: 2009).

parents responsible for their children's plight since they are the ones who brought them to this world, and receive benefits on their behalf (a child allowance), as in many advanced economies. Even if we hold parents responsible, two questions remain: One, to what extent should they sacrifice their individual liberties and the pursuit of their life goals for their children? Two, to what extent can we justifiably 'rely on the natural affection and goodwill of the mature family members' (Rawls 2008), and what if they somehow fail to take proper care of children, willingly or unwillingly, consciously or unconsciously? Being affectionate and possessing goodwill does not mean parents always know what is best for their children. Lack of parental education—not necessarily in a modern sense—is a critical determinant of child mortality. No wonder that libertarians like Friedman (1955) and Hayek (2013) too argue for state financing of children's education.

As far as individual rights are concerned, Rawls outlined a list of minimal and urgent human rights, like the right to life, which he regarded as a special class of rights that are universally applicable, and made a strong case for them by arguing that they 'specify limits to a regime's internal autonomy', and when that limit is trespassed, they provide and restrict 'the justifying reasons for war and its conduct' (Rawls 2008). However, he does not specifically talk of children's right to life, which has very different implications, empirical as well as normative, vis-à-vis an adult's right to life. Other political philosophers, too, have come out strongly in support of the right to life. Ayn Rand (1964: 89), for example, saw 'a man's right to his own life' as the 'only *one* fundamental right', and other rights as its consequences or corollaries. Although Michael Walzer (1983: 79) made a case in favour of culturally relative theories of justice as against 'a single formula, universally applicable', he made an even stronger pitch in favour of the universal individual rights to life and liberty.[27] For Walzer, like Rawls, these rights provide the justification for the right of states to territorial integrity and political sovereignty; when states fail to protect and promote them, external aggression against

---

[27] To him, 'how these rights are themselves founded I cannot try to explain here. It is enough to say that they are somehow entailed by our sense of what it means to be a human being. If they are not natural, then we have invented them, but natural or invented, they are a palpable feature of our moral world' (Walzer 2006: 54).

them is justified, the limits to which are set by these rights (Walzer 2006). However, none of them has particularly discussed children's right to life or other relevant rights.

The implications of not specifying a special right to life for children is visible in the proposals that have been made in connection with what it entails. For Rand (1964: 89–90), recognizing a person's right to life is tantamount to recognizing his 'right to engage in self-sustaining and self-generated action', his right to the fruits of his own efforts (that is, his right to property), and 'freedom from physical compulsion, coercion or interference by other men'. Nozick (1974: 179) argues that a 'supposed' right to life is, at best, 'a right to have or strive for whatever one needs to live', provided it does not violate anyone's rights, and that 'a theory of property rights' is the foundation on which a right to life should be erected. For Rawls (2008: 65), it seems to imply a right to the 'means of subsistence and security'; for Walzer (2004), 'a police force' and 'public health service', banning of 'child labor', passing of 'minimum wage laws', and so forth. Scanlon (1977: 92) sees the right to life 'as a complex of elements including particular liberties to act in one's own defense and to preserve one's life, claim rights to aid and perhaps to the necessities of life'. As is evident, children can neither engage in 'self-sustaining action' or 'strive' to fulfil their needs, nor can we stop at making it a positive right and making provisions for 'resources' of any kind, holding them responsible for the outcomes of using those resources. At the same time, their right to life cannot also mean a responsibility to save each and every child, because, no matter what we do, not all child deaths would be 'preventable'. As we will argue later, a child's right to life should be a right to the 'capability to avoid premature mortality', which is neither completely proceduralist nor consequentialist. Justice for children brings out the complexity of notions of both injustice and justice, the challenge of addressing them without well-reasoned argumentation and consideration.

Relevance of Sen's Approach to Justice

Sen's capability approach and idea of justice are a limited exception to the general tendencies in political philosophy as outlined above. Although Rawls has had an epochal impact not only on political philosophy and philosophers, but on the way justice is seen and argued today, and though he saw Sen's approach as an 'unworkable' idea which 'calls for more information than political society can conceivably acquire and sensibly apply' (Rawls 2008), Sen's approach has held sway over a wider academic terrain,[28] and has also provided the conceptual framework for a variety of indicators that try to reflect, even if partially, the actual human condition—the Human Development Index (HDI) of the United Nations Development Programme[29] (UNDP) and the Multidimensional Poverty Index (MPI) of the Oxford Poverty and Human Development Initiative (OPHI) being two cases.[30] His approach has also provided intellectual inspiration for the official poverty and wealth reports of the German government (Arndt and Volkert 2007), and there have been several efforts at its operationalization in various disciplines and contexts.

Sen introduced the notion of 'basic capabilities' in his Tanner Lecture (Sen 1979), and later went on to develop and apply his capability approach for the analysis of well-being, standard of living, economic inequality, poverty, development, freedom, gender bias, social justice, and so forth. The central premise of his approach is that humans are quite diverse in terms of their internal characteristics (such as age, sex, abilities and disabilities, talents, and proneness to illness) as well as external circumstances (social, economic, ecological, among others), and therefore their capabilities to convert a given set of resources,[31]

---

[28] See Robeyns (2005) for an interdisciplinary survey of the capability approach.

[29] See Fukuda-Parr (2003) for a discussion on the connections between Sen's approach and the Human Development Reports.

[30] See Clark (2006) and Robeyns (2006) for how capability approach has been put into practice.

[31] Even lack of resources or poverty is seen by Sen in terms of capability-deprivation (Sen 2000). Although the 'income-poverty' of a Dalit and an upper-caste person might be the same, but the 'capability-poverty' of a poor Dalit will most likely be higher than his UC counterpart due to their differential external characteristics. Nevertheless, it is also possible that the income-poor UC person has a higher level of capability-poverty due to his/her deprivations arising out of internal characteristics, or even external circumstances in certain cases. For instance, income-poor UC woman may quite possibly be more capability-deprived than an equally income-poor Dalit man, which is why Sen argues we need to move beyond resources to people's capabilities.

including Rawls's 'social primary goods', into valuable achievements also vary. Drawing on Aristotle's notions of 'highest good'[32] (which for Aristotle consists in *eudaimonia* or happiness) and 'human flourishing', as well as Marx's concept of 'commodity fetishism' (Marx 1982), Sen argues that the central focal variable should—unlike resourcist theories of justice, including that of Rawls—consist not of resources (means) we own, but of our capabilities to pursue ends we have reason to value. Capability refers to our substantive freedoms to choose from various combinations of valuable 'functionings' (doings and beings)—which can be as basic as being alive, in good health, adequately nourished, and so forth, to higher achievements such as being happy, participating in community-life, having self-respect, and so forth. The freedom to choose not only has instrumental value (to the extent it helps us in pursuing our ends), but an intrinsic value which directly contributes to our well-being (an important reason why capabilities, not functionings, should be the focal variable). Nevertheless, since reliable data on capabilities is not usually available, we have to rely on the functionings people are able to achieve. This is not always a problem, especially in the case of basic capabilities like capability to avoid premature mortality, because achievement in such cases tends to be a good guide to our underlying capabilities, for we usually prefer longer and healthier lives for ourselves, our families and children whenever we have the capability to do so (Sen 1985, 1999, 2000, 2002, 2003, 2006).

By moving the focus *beyond* means, the capability approach does not only accommodate and respect human diversity, but also cultural diversity, and that of a wide variety of means (in our context, determinants of child survival). The tribal case in India is very interesting. Better child survival among them was not a result of Western biomedicine—they were, and still are, farthest from it—and anthropologists like Verrier Elwin highlighted how Indian tribals were more better in many respects than Europeans and mainstream Indian population. Better child survival among tribals was the result not of any vaccinations, but of a social, economic and political system that was much more woman- and child-friendly. Among core elements of tribal life illustrated by Elwin were: 'identity with Nature,

---

[32] In *Nicomachean Ethics*, Aristotle argues that 'wealth is evidently not the good we are seeking; for it is merely useful and for the sake of something else' (Aristotle 1998: 7).

the honoured place of women ... the love of children, a strong sense of community and equality' (Guha 1996: 2377). According to Maharatna (2005), 'these admittedly admirable sociocultural features of Indian tribes have a bearing on and are largely corroborated by their demographic features and behaviour'. Nevertheless, as he further reflects, instead of learning from these tribal traits, the entire discourse has centred around how best they could be integrated into the 'mainstream'. Scholars have also highlighted the 'north-south sociocultural divide' in India, where the South is characterized by better female autonomy and sex ratio vis-à-vis the North, and has played a key role in demographic differentials between the two, not least child mortality (Basu 1992; Das Gupta 1987; Dyson and Moore 1983; Kishor 1993; Maharatna 2005).

The contextual nature of determinants (means) has been, to an extent, highlighted in the literature on determinants and models of child survival, albeit inadequately. Means are not limited to financial resources alone—in a great many cases, at least in the long run, removing barriers to people's development and prosperity would be an important area to focus on. It allows for variations in solutions at the local level, without indulging in any form of 'fetishism of the commodity', and allows space for a variety of models and aetiologies of child survival and health. It also helps understand the local variations in child mortality, without being pressured to explain all by means of the preferred space of means. The potential of those who could do better is also not left untapped by focusing exclusively on those who are actually not doing well. There is importance attached to the process aspect of freedom, although not in the form of a central focal variable, which would be a boost to aggregative efficiency too (as these people can contribute significantly to the overall decline with fewer resources compared to the ones who are not doing good and start from a lower point). In this sense, the capability approach would help in the design of a comprehensive child survival policy which incorporates the concerns of equity as well as efficiency. If we just focus on *equity* of an outcome type, we would only focus on those who are not doing well. If we only focus on *efficiency* of an outcome type, we may as well be putting our resources on those large groups which are capable of substantial reductions in child mortality at the aggregate level—and helping us achieve targets like MDG4 with fewer resources and quickly—than those who would need more resources and time. A focus on capability approach can also help in making accountability much more achievement-, rather than input-oriented, which has thankfully already started under the present Government of India.

As far as children are concerned, though Sen has not explicitly focused on them, his approach to 'freedom', which constitutes people's capabilities, justifies their inclusion within the scope of justice. Unlike Friedman (1955), for instance, who excludes 'irresponsible individuals' like children and the 'insane' from his concept of freedom, Sen makes a distinction between what he calls 'effective freedom' and 'freedom as control'. While the latter refers to the freedom of pursuing or achieving things that one values through the exercise of direct individual agency, the former is much more comprehensive inasmuch as it also includes freedoms afforded to us by the exercise of public agency or, indirectly, by the exercise of other individuals' agencies. The former is an integral feature of life in a society, especially that of a complex modern type, in which 'many freedoms'—for example, freedom from malaria and epidemics, freedom to move around safely, or even freedom to realize one's libertarian or other rights—are afforded to us 'without the levers of control being directly operated by us' (Sen 1995).

Although both types of freedoms are valued within the capability perspective, and are seen as contributing to well-being of rational adults ('choosing' has intrinsic as well as instrumental value, and contributes directly to well-being too), we can make assessments of justice among children—as well as among adults who are unable to exercise reasoned agency—starting with an exclusive focus on 'effective freedoms' enjoyed by them, and extend it to include 'choice' as they develop rational agency. Biggeri, Ballet, and Comim (2011: 4) make a case for seeing children 'as agents in the process of developing their capabilities and well-being', but this could only be argued as far as grown-up children are concerned, and not in the case of children under the age of five, with whom we are concerned in this book. In fact, responding to Cohen's charge that 'small babies do not sustain themselves through exercises of capability' (Cohen 1993a), Sen argued that 'athleticism was never intended', and though babies and the mentally disabled are not in a position to exercise reasoned 'active choice', we can still assess their capabilities (in terms of 'achieved functionings' [*doings* and *beings*, but only *beings* would be relevant in this case] and 'well-being achievement') through 'elementary evaluation' (equating the value of the capability set to the value of one of its elements). The characterization of the capability approach has to be related to the 'evaluative purpose' of the exercise in question (Sen 1993). One could argue that the lesser there is scope for 'active choice' within the sphere of capabilities, and 'doings' in that of functionings, the greater there is the need for enhancing the 'effective freedom' and 'beings' of concerned individuals through public action—as well as parental in the context of children.

Sen not only objected to Rawls's focal variable, but also the focus of theories of justice. He argued that our focus should be on the identification and removal of manifest and redressable injustices, and enhancing justice, rather than the characterization of a perfectly just society. In the assessment of justice, we need to focus on 'actual lives' people are able to lead instead of focusing on the basic structure of society and its institutions. He brings out the distinction between these two approaches by using two concepts from traditional Indian jurisprudence—the concept of *nyaya*, concerned in particular with lives that people are actually able to lead, and that of *niti*, relating to 'organizational propriety as well as behavioural correctness'. Likewise, he identifies two lines of thinkers of the Enlightenment period—one that focused on the 'social contract' and perfect justice (represented by Hobbes, Locke, Rousseau, Kant, and Rawls), the other on comparative justice, sharing an interest in comparisons of ways in which people may lead their lives (represented by Smith, Condorcet, Bentham, Marx, Mill, and Sen himself 'to a great extent'). With focus on actual lives, his approach concentrates on actual behaviour of people as well as other determinants of justice, instead of just assuming a strict compliance by all with requirements of perfect justice. It also needs to be pointed out that the focus on injustice does not imply a curative approach, and Sen does particularly talk about 'prevention of manifest injustice', and about prevention of famines—which, according to him, are not a case of misfortune, but that of injustice—many times in the same work.[33]

---

[33] Cahn also talked about prevention of injustice while defining justice as 'the active process of remedying or *preventing* what would arouse the "sense of injustice"' (Cahn 1966: 11, emphasis added), between the two extremes of justice as a static ideal and justice as merely a quality of human will or a good motive.

Prevention relates to not just social structure and institutions, but also non-institutional features (Sen 2009).

With his focus on 'real ends' (Sen 1995), 'actual lives', 'actual realizations', 'actual societies that would emerge', the role of 'non-institutional features' or the 'actual behaviours of people and their social interactions' in influencing the nature of the society, given any set of institutions (Sen 2009), and his proposal to make assessments based on 'comparative justice' (on the kinds of lives people could possibly lead), Sen's capability approach and idea of justice display a sensitivity to the real world that is lacking in other approaches to justice. He, in fact, undertook what he referred to as a 'case-implication critique'—analysing implications that a particular normative theory would have in the light of particular cases—and not just a 'prior-principle critique'—analysing the consistency of a principle based on abstract prior principles—of Rawlsian and utilitarian approaches to equality and justice in his Tanner Lecture of 1979.

Contextual Relevance of the Capability Approach[34]

With a focus on people's capabilities and 'actual lives', Sen's capability approach and idea of justice are particularly relevant for analysis of cases wherein discrimination, both 'direct' and 'structural', is pervasive and profoundly affects people's capabilities and life-chances. Few cases would be as befitting as India, if we take into account the entrenched nature of multiple, overlapping patterns of discrimination, even after close to seven decades of constitutional and institutional promises of equality and social justice. B.R. Ambedkar, Chairman of the Drafting Committee of India's Constitution, foresaw the inadequacy of *formal* justice—'It might have been thought that this principle of equal justice would strike a death blow to the Established Order. As a matter of fact, far from suffering any damage the Established Order has continued to operate in spite of it' (Ambedkar 1989: 103–4).

There is enough evidence to support Ambedkar's and Sen's scepticism towards formal justice. For instance, according to Drèze and

---

[34] This section has been reproduced from an earlier book of mine (Mehdi 2014).

Kingdon (2001: 20), 'scheduled-caste children have an "intrinsic disadvantage" in the sense of a relatively low chance of going to school even after controlling for household wealth, parental education and motivation, school quality, and related variables', suggesting 'persistence of an overall bias against scheduled-caste children in the schooling system, in spite of positive discrimination in pupil incentives'. Jeffrey, Jeffery, and Jeffery (2004) provide qualitative evidence regarding capability-deprivation of educated Dalits to convert their cultural capital into secure employment. A World Bank study highlighted that 'being an SC significantly lowers the probability of movement out of poverty even after we control for the effects of many other factors' (Kapoor et al. 2009). Lanjouw and Zaidi (2001) found out that not only are Dalit households deprived vis-à-vis asset ownership as well as human capital, they also experience lower economic returns from both. Dommaraju, Agadjanian, and Yabiku (2008: 491) argue that 'caste differentials in health outcomes such as child mortality cannot be reduced to socioeconomic differences among castes', pointing to the independent impact of caste discrimination. In the study by van de Poel and Speybroeck (2009: 282) on malnutrition inequalities between SC/STs and the remaining Indian population, they conclude that 'it is important to consider both differences in the distribution of health determinants and differences in their effects as the latter can point to behavioral differences or discriminatory behavior'. 'Behavioural differences' between groups such as SCs and UCs are themselves a result of 'discriminatory behaviour' that the former have been experiencing since centuries rather than of some essentialized genetic or cultural differences between them and other caste groups. One of the most important narratives of current Indian politics is around the *appeasement* of Muslims—invoking capability approach not only helps in analysing the reality of it, but also in helping us address it to an extent.

In the next chapter, we have a more detailed discussion of the proposed metrics of justice and how Sen's approach seems more suited as a conceptual framework to addressing child mortality. Their respective empirical relevance—based on data on child mortality and access to determinants of child survival, analysed in subsequent chapters—are discussed in the final chapter.

References

Ambedkar, B.R. 1989. *Dr. Babasaheb Ambedkar. Writings and Speeches*. Mumbai: Government of Maharashtra.

Aristotle. 1998. *The Nicomachean Ethics*. Edited by J.L. Ackrill and J.O. Urmson and translated by William David Ross. Oxford: Oxford Paperbacks.

Arndt, Christian and Jürgen Volkert. 2007. 'A Capability Approach for Official German Poverty and Wealth Reports: Conceptual Background and First Empirical Results'. IAW-Diskussionspapiere 27, Institut für Angewandte Wirtschaftsforschung (IAW), Tübingen, Germany.

Arneson, Richard. 1989. 'Equality and Equal Opportunity for Welfare'. *Philosophical Studies* 56(1): 77–93.

Barry, Brian M. 1989. *A Treatise on Social Justice*. Berkeley: University of California Press.

Basu, Alaka M. 1992. *Culture, the Status of Women, and Demographic Behaviour. Illustrated with the Case of India*. Oxford: Clarendon Press.

Bhalotra, Sonia, Christine Valente, and Arthur van Soest. 2010. 'Religion and Childhood Death in India'. In *Handbook of Muslims in India*, edited by Rakesh Basant and Abusaleh Shariff, 123–64. New Delhi: Oxford University Press.

Biggeri, Mario, Jérôme Ballet, and Flavio Comim, eds. 2011. *Children and the Capability Approach*. Houndmills, Basingstoke, Hampshire/New York: Palgrave Macmillan.

Bojer, Hilde. 2000. 'Children and Theories of Social Justice'. *Feminist Economics* 6(2): 23–39.

Cahn, Edmond. 1949. *The Sense of Injustice*. New York: New York University Press.

———. 1966. *Confronting Injustice. The Edmond Cahn Reader*. Edited by Lenore Cahn with general introduction and prefatory chapter notes by Norman Redlich. Boston: Little, Brown and Company.

Clark, David. 2006. 'Capability Approach'. In *The Elgar Companion to Development Studies*, edited by David Clark, 32–45. Cheltenham, UK: Edward Elgar Publishing Ltd.

Cohen, G.A. 1993a. 'Amartya Sen's Unequal World'. *Economic and Political Weekly* 28(40): 2156–60.

———. 1993b. 'Equality of What? On Welfare, Goods, and Capabilities'. In *The Quality of Life*, edited by Martha Nussbaum and Amartya Sen, 7–29. Oxford: Clarendon Press.

Daniels, Norman. 1985. *Just Health Care*. Cambridge [Cambridgeshire], New York: Cambridge University Press.

———. 2008. *Just Health: Meeting Health Needs Fairly*. Cambridge, New York: Cambridge University Press.

Daniels, Norman, Bruce P. Kennedy, and Ichiro Kawachi. 1999. 'Why Justice is Good for Our Health: The Social Determinants of Health Inequalities'. *Daedalus* 128(4): 215–51.

Das Gupta, Monica. 1987. 'Selective Discrimination against Female Children in Rural Punjab, India'. *Population and Development Review* 13(1): 77–100.

Deutsch, Morton. 1983. 'Current Social Psychological Perspectives on Justice'. *European Journal of Social Psychology* 13(3): 305–19.

Deutsch, Morton and Janice M. Steil. 1988. 'Awakening the Sense of Injustice'. *Social Justice Research* 2(1): 3–23.

Dommaraju, Premchand, Victor Agadjanian, and Scott Yabiku. 2008. 'The Pervasive and Persistent Influence of Caste on Child Mortality in India'. *Population Research and Policy Review* 27(4): 477–95.

Drèze, Jean and Geeta Gandhi Kingdon. 2001. 'School Participation in Rural India'. *Review of Development Economics* 5(1): 1–24.

Dubber, Markus. 2006. *The Sense of Justice. Empathy in Law and Punishment.* New York: New York University Press.

Dworkin, Ronald. 1981. 'What Is Equality? Part 2: Equality of Resources'. *Philosophy & Public Affairs* 10(4): 283–345.

———. 1985. *A Matter of Principle.* Cambridge, MA: Harvard University Press.

———. 2002. *Sovereign Virtue. The Theory and Practice of Equality.* Cambridge, MA and London: Harvard University Press.

Dyson, Tim and Mick Moore. 1983. 'On Kinship Structure, Female Autonomy, and Demographic Behavior in India'. *Population and Development Review* 9(1): 35–60.

Elster, Jon. 1995. 'The Empirical Study of Justice'. In *Pluralism, Justice, and Equality,* edited by David Miller and Michael Walzer, 81–98. Oxford [England], New York: Oxford University Press.

Faden, R.R. and M. Powers. 2008. 'Health Inequities and Social Justice'. *Bundesgesundheitsblatt—Gesundheitsforschung Gesundheitsschutz* 51(2): 151–7.

Friedman, Milton. 1955. 'The Role of Government in Education'. *Economics and the Public Interest* 2(2): 85–107.

Fukuda-Parr, S. 2003. 'The Human Development Paradigm: Operationalizing Sen's Ideas on Capabilities'. *Feminist Economics* 9(2–3): 301–17.

Graf, Gunter, Ramsay MacMullen, and Gottfried Schweiger. 2015. *The Wellbeing of Children. Philosophical and Social Scientific Approaches.* Warsaw: De Gruyter Open.

Geruso, Michael and Dean Spears. 2014. 'Sanitation and Health Externalities. Resolving the Muslim Mortality Paradox'. https://www.isid.ac.in/~pu/seminar/dean.pdf (accessed 25 January 2014).

Guha, Ramachandra. 1996. 'Savaging the Civilized: Verrier Elwin and the Tribal Question in Late Colonial India'. *Economic and Political Weekly* 31(35–36–37): 2375–89.

Habermas, Jürgen. 1996. *Between Facts and Norms. Contributions to a Discourse Theory of Law and Democracy.* Cambridge, MA: The MIT Press.

Hart, Caroline, Mario Biggeri, and Bernhard Babic, eds. 2015. *Agency and Participation in Childhood and Youth. International Applications of the Capability Approach in Schools and Beyond.* London: Bloomsbury.

Hayek, Friedrich. 2013. *Law, Legislation and Liberty. A New Statement of the Liberal Principles of Justice and Political Economy.* London: Routledge.

Heckman, James J. and Tim Kautz. 2013. 'Fostering and Measuring Skills: Interventions that Improve Character and Cognition'. National Bureau of Economic Research (NBER) Working Paper Series.

Horton, John. 2005. 'A Qualified Defence of Oakeshott's Politics of Scepticism'. *European Journal of Political Theory* 4(1): 23–36.

ICMR. 2007. *Health Research Policy—ICMR.* New Delhi: Indian Council of Medical Research.

IGME. 2011. *Levels and Trends in Child Mortality. Report 2011.* New York: Interagency Group for Child Mortality Estimation.

———. 2015. *Levels and Trends in Child Mortality. Report 2015.* New York: Interagency Group for Child Mortality Estimation.

Illich, Ivan. 1976. *Limits to Medicine. Medical Nemesis, the Expropriation of Health.* London: Boyars.

ILO. 2017. *Global Estimates of Child Labour. Results and Trends: 2012–2016.* Geneva: International Labour Organization.

Jeffrey, Craig, Roger Jeffery, and Patricia Jeffery. 2004. 'Degrees without Freedom: The Impact of Formal Education on Dalit Young Men in North India'. *Development and Change* 35(5): 963–86.

Kapoor, Soumya, Deepa Narayan, Saumik Paul, and Nina Badgaiyan. 2009. 'Caste Dynamics and Mobility in Uttar Pradesh'. In *Moving Out of Poverty*, edited by Deepa Narayan, Lant Pritchett, and Soumya Kapoor, 166–233. Washington, DC: The World Bank and Palgrave Macmillan.

Kazemi, Ali and Kjell Törnblom. 2008. 'Social Psychology of Justice: Origins, Central Issues, Recent Developments, and Future Directions'. *Nordic Psychology* 60(3): 209–34.

Kishor, Sunita. 1993. 'May God Give Sons to All: Gender and Child Mortality in India'. *American Sociological Review* 58(2): 247–65.

Kulkarni, P.M. 2010. 'The Muslim Population of India: A Demographic Portrayal'. In *Handbook of Muslims in India*, edited by Rakesh Basant and Abusaleh Shariff, 92–122. New Delhi: Oxford University Press.

Lanjouw, P. and S. Zaidi. 2001. *Determinants of Household Welfare in India.* World Bank Poverty Policy Note. Washington, DC: The World Bank.

Leßmann, Ortrud, Hans-Uwe Otto, and Holger Ziegler. 2011. *Closing the Capabilities Gap. Renegotiating Social Justice for the Young.* Opladen: Barbara Budrich.

Lipkus, Isaac M. 1992. 'A Heuristic Model to Explain Perceptions of Unjust Events'. *Social Justice Research* 5(4): 359–84.

Lötter, H.P.P. 1993. *Justice for an Unjust Society*. Value Inquiry Book Series. Amsterdam, Atlanta, GA: Rodopi.

Lucas, J.R. 1980. *On Justice. Peri dikaiou*. Oxford, NY: Clarendon Press; Oxford University Press.

Macleod, Colin. 2010. 'Primary Goods, Capabilities, and Children'. In *Measuring Justice*, edited by Harry Brighouse and Ingrid Robeyns, 174–92. Cambridge: Cambridge University Press.

Maharatna, Arup. 2005. *Demographic Perspectives on India's Tribes*. New Delhi: Oxford University Press.

Marx, Karl. 1982. *Capital*. Vol. 1 of *A Critique of Political Economy*. Translated by Ben Fowkes. Harmondsworth, England: Penguin Books.

McKeown, Thomas. 1979. *The Role of Medicine. Dream, Mirage, or Nemesis?* Princeton, NJ: Princeton University Press.

Mehdi, Ali. 2014. 'The Elusive Pursuit of Social Justice for Dalits in Uttar Pradesh'. In *Development Failure and Identity Politics in Uttar Pradesh*, edited by Roger Jeffery, Craig Jeffrey, and Jens Lerche, 75–103. New Delhi: SAGE.

Mikula, G. 1984. 'Justice and Fairness in Interpersonal Relations: Thoughts and Suggestions'. In *The Social Dimension*, edited by Henri Tajfel, 204–27. Cambridge: Cambridge University Press.

Mikula, Gerold, Birgit Petri, and Norbert Tanzer. 1990. 'What People Regard as Unjust: Types and Structures of Everyday Experiences of Injustice'. *European Journal of Social Psychology* 20(2): 133–49.

Mill, John Stuart. 1998. *Utilitarianism (Oxford Philosophical Texts)*. Edited by Roger Crisp. Oxford: Oxford University Press.

Miller, D. 1991. 'Recent Theories of Social Justice'. *British Journal of Political Science* 21(3): 371–91.

MoHFW. 2016. *National Health Profile (NHP) of India—2016*. New Delhi: Central Bureau of Health Intelligence, Ministry of Health and Family Welfare (MoHFW), Government of India.

Moore, Barrington. 1978. *Injustice. The Social Bases of Obedience and Revolt*. UK: Palgrave Macmillan.

Nadda, Jagat Prakash. 2015. 'So Our Children May Live'. *The Times of India* 28 April.

Navarro, Vicente and Leiyu Shi. 2001. 'The Political Context of Social Inequalities and Health'. *Social Science & Medicine* 52(3): 481–91.

Nozick, Robert. 1974. *Anarchy, State, and Utopia*. Oxford and Cambridge, MA: Blackwell.

Okin, Susan Moller. 1989. *Justice, Gender, and the Family*. New York: Basic Books.

Panini, M.N. 2000. 'M N Srinivas and Sociology'. *Economic and Political Weekly* 35(4): 174–7.

Plato. 2003. *The Republic*. Translated with an introduction by Desmond Lee. London: Penguin.

Ramani, K.V., Dileep Mavalankar, Sanjay Joshi, Imran Malek et al. 2010. *Why Should 5000 Children Die in India Every Day? Major Causes and Managerial Challenges*. Ahmedabad: Indian Institute of Management.

Rand, Ayn. 1964. *The Virtue of Selfishness*. New York: Penguin.

Rawls, John. 1963. 'The Sense of Justice'. *The Philosophical Review* 72(3): 281–305.

———. 1971. *A Theory of Justice*. Cambridge, MA and London: The Belknap Press of Harvard University Press.

———. 1981. *The Basic Liberties and Their Priority. The Tanner Lecture on Human Values*. Michigan: The University of Michigan.

———. 1985. 'Justice as Fairness: Political Not Metaphysical'. *Philosophy & Public Affairs* 14(3): 223–51.

———. 1987. 'The Idea of an Overlapping Consensus'. *Oxford Journal of Legal Studies* 7(1): 1–25.

———. 1988. 'The Priority of Right and Ideas of the Good'. *Philosophy & Public Affairs* 17(4): 251–76.

———. 1989. 'The Domain of the Political and Overlapping Consensus'. *New York University Law (NYUL) Review* 64(2): 233–55.

———. 2001. *Justice as Fairness. A Restatement*. Cambridge, MA / London: The Belknap Press of Harvard University Press.

———. 2008. *The Law of Peoples. With 'The Idea of Public Reason Revisited'*. New Delhi: Universal Law Publishing.

RGI. 1983. *Survey on Infant and Child Mortality, 1979*. New Delhi: Office of the Registrar General of India, Ministry of Home Affairs, Government of India.

———. 1989. *Mortality Differentials in India, 1984*. New Delhi: Office of the Registrar General of India, Ministry of Home Affairs, Government of India.

Robeyns, Ingrid. 2005. 'The Capability Approach: A Theoretical Survey'. *Journal of Human Development* 6(1): 93–114.

———. 2006. 'The Capability Approach in Practice'. *Journal of Political Philosophy* 14(3): 351–76.

Roemer, John. 1996. *Theories of Distributive Justice*. Cambridge, MA: Harvard University Press.

Ruger, Jennifer. 2009. *Health and Social Justice*. New York: Oxford University Press.

Samaddar, Ranbir. 2009. *State of Justice in India: Issues of Social Justice*. New Delhi: SAGE.

Sen, Amartya. 1979. *Equality of What?* The Tanner Lecture on Human Values. Stanford: Stanford University.

———. 1985. *Commodities and Capabilities*. Amsterdam: North-Holland (Elsevier Science).

———. 1993. 'Capability and Well-being'. In *The Quality of Life*, edited by Martha Nussbaum and Amartya Sen, 30–53. Oxford: Clarendon Press.

———. 1995. *Inequality Reexamined*. New York: Russell Sage Foundation; Cambridge, MA: Harvard University Press.

———. 1999. 'Critical Reflection: Health in Development'. *Bulletin of the World Health Organization* 77(8): 619–23.

———. 2000. *Development as Freedom*. New York: Anchor Books.

———. 2002. 'Why Health Equity?' *Health Economics* 11(8): 659–66.

———. 2003. 'Development as Capability Expansion'. In *Readings in Human Development: Concepts, Measures and Policies for a Development Paradigm*, edited by Sakiko Fukuda-Parr and A.K. Shiva Kumar. New Delhi and New York: Oxford University Press.

———. 2006. 'Health Achievement and Equity: External and Internal Perspectives'. In *Public Health, Ethics and Equity*, edited by Sudhir Anand, Fabienne Peter, and Amartya Sen, 263–8. Oxford: Oxford University Press.

———. 2009. *The Idea of Justice*. Cambridge, MA: The Belknap Press of Harvard University Press.

Scanlon, T.M. 1977. 'Rights, Goals, and Fairness'. *Erkenntnis* 11(1): 81–95.

Shaw, George Bernard. 1909. *The Doctor's Dilemma. Preface on Doctors*. World eBook Library PGCC Collection, Project Gutenberg.

Shklar, Judith. 1990. *The Faces of Injustice*. New Haven: Yale University Press.

Simon, Thomas W. 1995. *Democracy and Social Injustice. Law, Politics, and Philosophy (Studies in Social and Political Philosophy)*. Lanham, MD and London: Rowman & Littlefield Publishers.

United Nations General Assembly. 1989. *Convention on the Rights of the Child*. http://www.un.org/documents/ga/res/44/a44r025.htm (accessed 21 February 2017).

UNPD. 2017. World Population Prospects: The 2017 Revision. Key Findings and Advance Tables. New York: Department of Economic and Social Affairs (DESA), Population Division.

van de Poel, Ellen and Niko Speybroeck. 2009. 'Decomposing Malnutrition Inequalities between Scheduled Castes and Tribes and the Remaining Indian Population'. *Ethnicity & Health* 14(3): 271–87.

Venkatapuram, Sridhar. 2011. *Health Justice. An Argument from the Capabilities Approach*. Cambridge: Polity.

Walzer, Michael. 1983. *Spheres of Justice. A Defense of Pluralism and Equality*. New York: Basic Books.

———. 2004. 'The Argument about Humanitarian Intervention'. In *Ethics of Humanitarian Interventions*, edited by Georg Meggle, 21–35. Heusenstamm: Ontos Verlag.

Walzer, Michael. 2006. *Just and Unjust Wars. A Moral Argument with Historical Illustrations*. New York: Basic Books.

Williams, Alan. 1997. 'Intergenerational Equity: An Exploration of the "Fair Innings" Argument'. *Health Economics* 6(2): 117–32.

Wolgast, Elizabeth H. 1987. *The Grammar of Justice*. Ithaca, New York: Cornell University Press.

2

Metrics of Justice

According to Amartya Sen (1995a), almost every moral theory of social arrangements that has stood the test of time demands equality or equal consideration in some 'space' considered central by it. While this demand may not be a logical necessity, it is difficult to imagine how a theory could achieve moral or social plausibility without incorporating impartiality and universality at some level. On analysing this in detail, it turns out that even those who consider themselves anti-egalitarian conceive of equality, implicitly, in terms of a particular space, and provide direct or indirect support to equal consideration of all within the space central to their theory. For instance, even if utilitarians do not support the equal enjoyment of utilities, they attach equal importance to the utility gains of every person. Libertarians are opposed to equality of utilities, incomes, and other things, but they do argue for equality of libertarian rights. Neither is the justification of inequalities in certain spheres, regarded as peripheral, ethically or socially tenable without supporting equality in an alternative sphere viewed as central—that is, 'the strategy of justifying inequality through equality', as Sen (1995a: 21) puts it—nor is the demand for equality in a specific focal space justifiable without the tolerance of possible inequalities in other spaces considered as peripheral within a theory. In this sense, every major moral theory of social arrangements is egalitarian in some fundamental respect, and possibly anti-egalitarian in other respects.

'Equality of What?'

So, for Sen, the primary question and point of dispute—obviously not the only one though—in the analysis of equality is not whether there is a need for equality or equal consideration of all, but, as he famously formulated it in his 1979 Tanner Lecture, 'Equality of What?'. 'In fact, equality, as an abstract idea, does not have much cutting power, and the real work begins with the specification of what it is that is to be equalized' across individuals in a just society (Anand, Peter, and Sen 2006). Which is the most plausible space in which we should demand equality? Sen has used this question as a 'classificatory principle', a 'device', as 'a general methodological approach', to evaluate some of the major ethical theories in terms of their chosen space, the 'evaluative space'—utilitarianism's 'utility', Rawls' 'social primary goods', Nozick's 'libertarian rights', Dworkin's 'bundle of resources', Cohen's 'midfare'—as well as argue for his preferred space of 'capabilities'. If a preferred variable is accepted as plausible in the 'egalitarian calculus', it could also be seen as relevant for other 'social calculus', including assessment of aggregative efficiency, as we also have to address the issue of the 'efficiency of what?' (Sen 1993)—a central concern together with equity and justice which, again, only Sen seems to have focused on.[1] While we may want to assign priority to equity and justice, as Rawls does unequivocally—'justice is the first virtue of social institutions', as he states in Chapter 1 of his magnum opus, *A Theory of Justice*—a simultaneous, or even a prior, concern for efficiency may mean higher aggregate growth and development and, likewise, a higher bar for equity. There has to be higher aggregate growth, and that higher growth has to be equitable. Nevertheless,

---

[1] For Sen, equality is not the only goal and concern of public policy. It has to be tackled along and balanced with the requirements of aggregative demands and efficiency (Sen 2008b: 2009), the absence of which 'can lead to severe curtailment of the capabilities that people can altogether have' (Sen 1995a: 8). Therefore, 'to deny the existence of the efficiency problem would be a great mistake' (Sen 1995b: 270) that may come in the way of serving the cause of equality or justice in the practical world. To reduce inequities or injustices, 'what is needed is a serious analysis of the feasibility of alternative arrangements that can be less iniquitous but no less efficient' (Sen 1995b: 270).

equity and justice have to be essential constituents of the very process of aggregative growth rather than concerns to be dealt with post-growth through some redistributive mechanism. This is one of the reasons why we need to consider these twin concerns simultaneously, and prefer a central focal variable that can be seen as relevant for both the egalitarian and the growth calculus.

Human Diversity and Flourishing

From Sen's perspective, the practical importance of the focal questions arises from the basic fact of pervasive human diversity in terms of internal characteristics (age, gender, abilities, talents, proneness to illness, and so on) as well as external circumstances (social and economic background, environmental conditions, and so on) so that equality in one space tends to conflict with equality in other spaces. For example, as a result of human heterogeneity (and that of choices), equality in terms of resources would, almost certainly, lead to unequal outcomes. On the other hand, equality in the space of desired outcomes would require an unequal distribution of relevant resources based on people's respective internal and external situations. The notion of equality is confronted by human diversity—by no means a trivial consideration, to be dealt with after the central principles of justice have been worked out with 'normal' individuals in mind—as well as with the plurality of spaces in terms of which it can be judged, highlighting the centrality of the question, equality of what?[2] Sen criticizes the argument of primordial equality—that 'all men are born equal'—as it overlooks human diversity, and can, therefore, be 'deeply inegalitarian', since different individuals may require different treatments to achieve, let us say, a basic level of well-being. Neither are individuals born equal—naturally or socially—nor can we equalize treatment across individuals based on any focal

[2] There are other issues on which ethical theories differ. For instance, Sen points out that the way the chosen space is utilized—the problem of 'appropriate indices' in the measurement of inequality—is a further point of dispute, but we are concerned here primarily with the choice of space and the implications that it will have for a child survival policy.

variable ignoring pervasive human diversity.[3] However, since human diversity 'can be hard to accommodate adequately in the usual evaluative framework', it has often been left 'substantially unaddressed in the evaluative literature' (Sen 1995a: 28).

The justification for Sen's emphasis on the focal variable being sensitive to pervasive human diversity comes from his view that resources in general have instrumental value, to the extent they help people in leading free and flourishing lives. Although Sen was not aware of them at the time of proposing his approach (1993), Martha Nussbaum (1987), another influential theorist of the capability approach, later pointed out to similarities between Aristotelian views on 'human flourishing', as the ultimate end of political activity,[4] and the capability approach. Sen later acknowledged not only the Aristotelian, but also the Confucian as well as Buddhist, motivational connections of his approach (Sen 2006a). Aristotle started out his *Nicomachean Ethics* (1996) by arguing that 'every art and every investigation, and likewise every practical pursuit or undertaking, seems to aim at some good ... for instance, the end of the science of medicine is health'. Certain ends become means to other ends, and since it will be 'futile and vain' if this process were to continue 'ad infinitum', there has to be 'one ultimate end', 'the supreme good', 'which we wish for its own sake, while we wish the others only for the sake of this' (Aristotle 1996). In section 5, Aristotle (cited in Nussbaum 1987) states that 'clearly wealth is not the good we are in search of, for it is only good as being useful, a means

---

[3] 'The demands of substantive equality can be particularly exacting and complex when there is a good deal of antecedent inequality to counter' (Sen 1995a: 1). 'Antecedent inequality' is reflected in certain internal characteristics (abilities, talents, proneness to illness, etc.)—which come to be seen as 'natural' or 'innate' over time (for instance, the historically acquired 'superiority' of privileged groups as well as the historically acquired 'inferiority' of discriminated groups)—and quite clearly in terms of people's external circumstances. One fundamental question is: what should be the starting historical point for justice and equality?

[4] In *Politics*, Aristotle (quoted in Nussbaum 1987: 2–3) says that 'it is evident that the best *politeia* is that arrangement according to which anyone whatsoever might do best and live a flourishing life', and that 'it is the job of the excellent lawgiver to consider ... how they will partake in the flourishing living (eudaemonia) that is possible for them'.

to something else', a theme that he consistently highlights throughout his *Politics*. In section 4, he tells us that most ordinary as well as refined people see this ultimate good as 'eudaimonia' [*sic*]—which, according to Sen, has often been 'misleadingly translated' simply as 'happiness', and should rather be seen as 'fulfilment of life' or 'human flourishing' (Sen 2003). In section 9, Aristotle further states 'that the greatest and noblest of all things should be left to fortune would be too contrary to the fitness of things', thereby infusing activity in the attainment of human flourishing, the suitable conditions for which have to be provided by the State. However, because of this approach, Aristotle sees children and animals as incapable of eudaemonia (Aristotle 1996). Sen points out that Aristotle also used the Greek word '*dunamin*', sometimes translated as 'potentiality', but which can also be taken to mean 'capability of existing or acting' (Sen 1993). Nevertheless, it needs to be noted that, despite similarities, there are differences in Aristotle's and Sen's approach to capabilities.[5]

Beyond Resources

Sen appears to argue that the metric of justice should be sensitive to the attainment of the ultimate end of human flourishing—as well as to its various constituents, like being able to avoid premature mortality, being healthy, and so on—and take into account the fact of human diversity in achieving that end. It is on the basis of these two premises that he seems to undertake a critique of various metrics of justice and propose his own capability approach. However, it is important to note here that the capability approach does not completely rule out any concern for most other metrics, but does not assign them a central position. Sen, for instance, does not underplay the derivative and instrumental value of incomes, wealth, commodities, or other resources. Rather, he argues that we have to look *beyond* them in order to understand deprivation and injustice in a richer and more fulsome way. No matter what focal variable we choose for assessing poverty, inequality, and injustice, for Sen (2006a), 'there will almost always be room for discriminating use of incomes and income-related statistics,

---

[5] For an elaborate discussion, see Nussbaum (1987).

particularly in explaining major deprivations related to economic causes'. As 'personal income is certainly a basic determinant even of survival and death, and more generally of the quality of life', he does not argue that traditional economic indicators should be completely abandoned, rather they should be supplemented with an 'epistemically rich' outlook, since, after all, 'income is only one variable among many that affect our chances of enjoying life' (Sen 1998).[6] Likewise, in judging a country's development, we cannot ignore the critical role of economic growth, but 'must look well beyond it' (Sen 2008a). One of Sen's primary contributions has been to motivate the conceptualization of development beyond its resourcist framework, in which human diversity and ends are neglected.

Accepting their derivative role, he argues that commodities possess various characteristics or properties, but unless we duly take into account the internal and external characteristics of the individual who has to use them and his ends,[7] it would be premature to arrive at any judgement about their use-value as far as that particular individual is concerned. A bicycle, for instance, possesses characteristics of transportation, but may not have use-value for a crippled person, while it could be highly valuable for an individual who does not suffer from that disability. Likewise, an individual may fail to be adequately nourished if he is suffering from a parasitic disease that makes the absorption of nutrients difficult, although the same amount of nutrients could be sufficient for another individual not affected such (Sen 1985). Since the focus of justice should be on human beings, and many, if not all, of them differ in terms of their internal and external characteristics, we have to look at the instrumental or use-value of commodities for the achievement of ends that are valuable in themselves.

Sen mentions two strategies for obtaining information on the quality of life that individuals are able to enjoy—(*a*) 'direct assessment' which takes into account their survival, health, education and other aspects

---

[6] In talking about the failures of entitlements during famines, Sen (2006a: 33) states that 'a fuller understanding of the pattern of deprivation and its distribution over the population requires us to go beyond the food availability statistics (while taking due note of them)'.

[7] 'Since means are ultimately valued for something else, it is not easy to set up a scheme of valuation of means that would be really independent of the ends' (Sen 1995a: 80).

of life; and (*b*) 'indirect appraisal' which considers their command over resources (based on the assumption that they are of equal use-value for all individuals). The first strategy is a 'radical departure' from 'conventional economics', and while 'there is clearly much to be gained from the interaction of the two approaches', we need to realize that they are fundamentally different in terms of the evaluative space that they view as suitable for assessing human advantage. Sen (1995c) adopts the first one, without denying the derivative relevance of the second. Issues which directly constitute a person's quality of life should have priority over those that play an instrumental role.

Any set of resources—either Rawls' 'social primary goods', Dworkin's 'bundle of resources', or any other—cannot, therefore, be a suitable metric of justice, since: (*a*) resources are merely 'means', and not valuable per se;[8] (*b*) different individuals would need different combinations of resources in different measures to achieve an optimal flourishing. As a result of advocating equality of some set of resources, not only do these theories suffer from a 'fetishist handicap' or 'commodity fetishism' (Sen draws inspiration from Marx as well), they would actually end up doing injustice to those who need greater resources to achieve a particular set of ends. A pregnant woman, a newborn baby, and an old or disabled person, would usually require greater healthcare and other resources than a healthy individual to survive and to lead healthy and flourishing lives. Especially in situations where we need to counter substantial 'antecedent inequality', this consideration would be of great significance, for equalizing the substantive and real opportunities individuals can enjoy.

---

[8] According to Sen (1995c: 20), 'it is good to have a high quality of life despite low income per head, but ultimately we have to be concerned not so much with achieving *high quality of life vis-a-vis income*, but with achieving *high quality of life*, full stop' (emphasis as per original). Quality of life can be enhanced by raising incomes per head ('growth-mediated development'), or by means of focusing on human development ('security-led development'). However, we also need to be concerned about rise in incomes as they help in pursuing various well-being and agency objectives. He mentions Kerala as a case, and argues that while its 'experience shows that even a very poor economy can have high achievement in quality of life through well-designed public policy', we also need to ask why incomes have not risen there (Sen 1995c: 20–1). Perhaps because of this one-sided development, he thinks it simplistic to see Kerala as a 'model'.

Beyond Utilities

Utilitarianism has been the dominant theory in ethical philosophy as well as standard welfare economics[9] for much of the modern era. Though it still seems to have a fair deal of influence in the latter realm, it stands thoroughly discredited in the former, thanks to the systematic and sustained critiques presented by a number of political philosophers, starting with Rawls. It has been criticized on many counts, but one of the most basic criticisms has been its distribution-indifference—or lack of concern for equity due to its principal efficiency orientation, reflected in its primary focus on the maximization of the sum total of utilities—though it is said to have had a historically 'radical role in providing effective critiques of many traditional inequities', which could also be seen as thoroughly inefficient. Nonetheless, as its concern with inequities is only indirect and peripheral at best, it cannot be an adequate theory of justice (Sen 1995a).

Beyond its problematic 'focal combination' of utility summation and maximization, Sen (2000a) has also criticized its 'basal space' or its mental metric of happiness or pleasure as the primary focal variable for assessment of justice for a variety of reasons. One, such a metric is not sensitive to human flourishing and well-being. People adapt to their circumstances and try to draw happiness or pleasure with whatever they are or have, when it does not seem realistic to them to desire those things or ends that are not possible within their given situation. This is especially so in the case of entrenched inequalities, when adaptation appears to be the best strategy of satisfying survival.[10] Happiness or desires are highly subjective metrics and cannot, therefore, be considered

---

[9] In standard welfare economics, utilitarianism has been used to assess individual well-being in terms of utilities enjoyed by people, usually in the form of happiness or desire fulfilment. However, as it is difficult to directly measure the mental metrics of happiness and desire, the ownership of commodities is used as a proxy to assess people's achievement of these metrics (Sen 1995b). We have already discussed earlier the limitations of relying on commodities for the assessment of well-being.

[10] Conversely, they may also feel unhappy or unfulfilled even when they are able to lead flourishing lives which are optimally possible for them or within the parameters of their society.

as reliable guides for human well-being and flourishing. 'Basing the assessment of justice on a measuring rod that bends and twists and adapts as much as utilities do, can be formidably problematic' (Sen 1995b: 263). Two, happiness and the fulfilment of pleasure or desire are *one* dimension of well-being, and we cannot *primarily* focus on them ignoring other more fundamental and critical dimensions of well-being. Three, these metrics do not take into account processes through which people achieve their utilities or freedoms enjoyed by them. 'This informational neglect' applies both to overall or positive freedoms as well as to negative freedoms (Sen 2000a). Lastly, but significantly, human diversity is ignored, assuming 'everyone gets the same utility from the same commodity basket' (Sen 2000a), along with a focus on commodities or resources.

However, Sen (1979) has made an attempt 'to provide a critique of utilitarianism without disputing the acceptability of consequentialism'. He argues that there is no essential link between consequentialism and welfarism. The 'goodness of states of affairs' can be assessed based on consequentialist considerations other than welfarist utility, which could be of intrinsic value—such as well-being and flourishing. Consequences are an important consideration. To have an overall assessment of justice, it is crucial to look not only at actions, but their various consequences for intrinsically valuable end states. 'To ignore consequences is to leave an ethical story half told'. Third, he makes a distinction between consequentialism and consequentialist reasoning—the former demands 'that the rightness of actions be judged entirely by the goodness of consequences', while the latter involves taking consequences into consideration without ignoring procedural or other considerations (Sen 2004: 75). Like utilitarianism, the capability approach too is an instance of 'outcome morality', but not in an exclusivist sense, since it also takes into account the processes and the freedoms by means of which 'diverse' people achieve certain outcomes.

As far as the specific issue of child survival is concerned, the utilitarian metric of happiness, desire, or pleasure appears to have no direct relevance. We first need to be alive before we can either be happy or be able to fulfil our desires or pleasures, and utilitarianism does not seem to provide any normative proposal—direct or indirect—that could ensure the survival and well-being of children. Their survival would be relevant for the happiness and desire-fulfilment of their parents, and since most theories of justice regard children as the responsibility of their parents, without taking into consideration children themselves—as they are not full citizens yet—it would not be surprising if utilitarianism were to focus on happiness or desire-fulfilment of the former rather than the survival and well-being of the latter. However, if consequentialism is an exclusive focus on consequences of actions, then it does seem relevant in the case of children too (their survival and health), although the same cannot be said about the utility metric per se. However, as we discuss later, there is a scope, although limited, for freedom here as well.

Beyond Libertarian Rights

Systematic libertarian theories like the one proposed by Nozick (1974) have, unlike the 'bends and twists' of the utilitarian 'measuring rod', argued for a rigid focus on liberties and rights as constitutive of the basal space or central focal variable. 'Individuals have rights, and there are things no person or group may do to them.... So strong and far-reaching are these rights that they raise the question of what, if anything, the state and its officials may do' (1974: xix). General libertarian critiques of utilitarianism and egalitarianism had existed for long, but with the emergence of well worked out libertarian theories, a focus on liberties and rights was enunciated much more sharply, and exclusively, unlike Hayek and other libertarians. 'No trade-offs are permitted' (Sen 1979: 214). The 'judgments are not of the "more-or-less" kind, but of the "zero-one" type' (Sen 2000a). Additionally, all such rights are negative rights and the most we can expect is protection by the State against their violation. These rights cannot be overridden by other concerns, and it is only when they have been fulfilled can there be scope for any other concern. Since trade-offs in terms of these rights are not allowed, no matter how much human misery is produced or coexists with the fulfilment of these rights—'even famines can result without anyone's libertarian rights being violated', as Sen (2000a) counter-argues—this focal space seems inhumanly restricted and extremist, and cannot, therefore, form the basis of an appropriate theory of justice. Not only does it ignore human flourishing, it does not seem to make space for human diversity. However, libertarianism, unlike utilitarianism, is equity-sensitive inasmuch as it gives equal weight to the rights and liberties of all individuals, without any considerations of aggregative efficiency being allowed to compromise with the fulfilment of anyone's libertarian rights, as Nozick's categorical statement demonstrates. However, before we end here, we need to admit and acknowledge that there is a lot of diversity of views within the libertarian framework and we have tried to restrict ourselves to the most central and relevant aspects of it from the perspective of our concern with child survival.

Equality of Capabilities

Since the phrase 'capability theory of justice' (Alexander 2010) has been used, it needs to be clarified at the outset that, unlike several of its competitors, Sen's capability approach is *not* a full theory of justice—it only pertains to the dimension of the focal variable, the basal space, based on which assessments of justice and injustice should be made, and a rejection of other spaces on which they should not be. Sen (1995b) had clarified—'I have not gone beyond outlining a space and some general features of a combining formula, and this obviously falls far short of being a complete theory of justice'. However, in his more comprehensive and relatively newer work, *The Idea of Justice* (Sen 2009: ix), he does claim to present 'a theory of justice in a very broad sense'. We discuss relevant dimensions of it after a brief discussion of his metric of justice.

In contrast to the metrics discussed earlier, Sen has argued for an 'informationally rich evaluative framework' (Sen 2000a) that is characterized by '*internal* plurality' (Sen 1995a; emphasis as per original)[11]

---

[11] The capability approach, being a complex approach, unlike most of its competitors, argues against the 'arbitrary requirement of descriptive homogeneity', and supports a 'multiplicity of ethically valuable considerations' (Sen 2004: 61–2). Sen (1985: 2) thinks that 'formal economics has not been very interested in the plurality of focus in judging a person's states and interests', and has rather often seen the 'richness of the subject matter' as an 'embarrassment', and has therefore been obsessed with reducing it to a simple single variable. However, 'given the variety of contexts in which the assessment of interest is relevant, it is quite unlikely that we shall get some one measure of interest that is superior to all others and applicable in all contexts'. His purpose is, thus, 'not the search for such a magic measure', but 'more to clarify the roles and limitations of different concepts of interest, and to fill in what may well be important gaps in the conceptual apparatus of interest-assessment and the judgment of advantage and well-being' (Sen 1985: 7).

and is sensitive to 'comprehensive outcomes'—processes, freedoms, achievements, and so on—not just to 'means' (as resourcist variables are), or only to 'simple' or 'culmination' outcomes (as the utilitarian metric is), followed by an arbitrary dismissal of all other concerns (Sen 2009). Pervasive human diversity complicates the unifocal pursuit of equality in a narrow space, ignoring considerations of equality in other spaces, or demands of efficiency and other important considerations (2009: 295–6). However, Sen seems to have occasionally argued in favour of equality of 'freedom' (Sen 1995a), of 'freedoms' (1995a: xi, 80, 151; Sen 2000a: 72n18), 'overall freedoms' (Sen 1995a), 'substantive freedoms' (1995a: 33), 'effective freedoms' (1995a: 86), 'capabilities' (or 'the elimination of unambiguous inequalities in capabilities')[12] (1995a: 7), of 'capability and substantive freedom' (Sen 2009), and so on—without conferring an absolutist status on either of these possibilities. In fact Sen (2009: 295) asks whether it would 'be right to presume that we should demand equality *of* capability', and responds in the negative. Let us briefly consider relevant concepts in the capability approach and see how justice is to be judged within its framework.

Freedom

Freedom is the broadest concern in Sen's framework. According to him, it is the ultimate aim of public policy, of development, to enhance

---

[12] Sen's focus on elimination of unambiguous capability inequities appears in sync with his recent priority to the removal of manifest and redressable injustices (Basu and Kanbur 2009; Sen 2009). It is perhaps of some significance that his book in which he systematically dealt with the question, 'equality of what?', was titled, *Inequality Reexamined* (Sen 1995a), and not 'Equality' Reexamined. Perhaps, it would have been more appropriate to even frame the question as, 'inequality of what?', in line with his focus on inequality and injustice, but maybe he did not do it since other theories focus on equality, not inequality. However, it also seems to be the case that the focus on inequality or injustice was not as developed in his earlier works as in *The Idea of Justice* (Sen 2009), in which he has forcefully argued the case for focusing on the elimination of manifest and redressable injustices rather than on 'perfect justice'.

people's 'substantive freedoms',[13] to remove manifest 'unfreedoms', so that they can pursue ends that they have reason to value. Unless we have necessary freedoms, we cannot be held responsible for the choices that we make or the consequences that we face (Sen 2008b). Freedom is not only the 'primary end' of development, it is also its 'principal means'—political and civil freedoms, for instance, are not only *intrinsically* valuable, they also *instrumentally* help us to influence public policy for the enhancement of substantive freedoms. Sen argues that his perspective of freedom has linkages with the writings of not only libertarian thinkers like Hayek, Nozick, Buchanan, and others, but also with that of Marx—concerned as he was with 'the conditions of the free development and movement of individuals' (Sen 1995a: 41n8; Marx and Engels 1998: 89). Sen's approach, however, seems more in sync with the latter since he valued freedom ultimately for intrinsic reasons, going way beyond its instrumental relevance (Sen 1988: 271).

Opportunity and Process Freedom

Freedom has 'two different and irreducibly diverse aspects'—the 'opportunity aspect' and the 'process aspect' (Sen 2002c). The former relates to 'real' opportunities people possess to achieve ends that they have reason to value, which may not necessarily be related to one's well-being, and may even involve ends which limit or undermine it. The process aspect of freedom corresponds to 'the *processes* that allow freedom of actions and decisions', such as resources, political and civil rights, and liberties (Sen 2008b; emphasis as per original). This 'process aspect' appears to be related to the 'means' of freedom, and it is not necessary that it enables one to achieve the 'opportunity aspect' of freedom. Both aspects of freedom are important for the assessment of justice and concentration on the former does not imply a neglect of the latter. One might want to have freedom to achieve an end, and also want to achieve it with fair means or procedures. For Sen (1995a: 87), 'if our concern is with

---

[13] It is possible that not all sorts of freedoms are valued, and some might even be seen as a burden, either because they may be trivial or impose unwanted responsibilities, loss of time and energy, which might be used for better ends (Sen 1995a). It seems, therefore, that Sen is concerned with 'substantive freedoms', not with all of them.

equality of freedom, it is no more adequate to ask for equality of its *means* than it is to seek equality of its *results*. Freedom relates to both, but does not coincide with either' (emphasis as per original).

Well-being and Agency Freedom

As the opportunity aspect of freedom may or may not be related to one's well-being, Sen made a further distinction between 'well-being freedom' (relating to 'well-being objectives') and 'agency freedom' (relating to the more comprehensive 'agency objectives', which may or may not include or give priority to one's 'well-being objectives'). Likewise, he distinguishes between 'well-being achievement' and 'agency achievement', and argues that there may not necessarily be a congruence between the two types of freedoms and achievements, or across them. It is quite possible that agency freedom leads to a reduction in well-being freedom and well-being achievement. For instance, one might pursue a charitable work for the well-being of others that leads to the curtailment of one's own well-being freedom and achievement, and although the agency freedom is exercised in this case, it is not certain whether this will lead to agency achievement as well. Similarly, well-being freedom does not always lead to well-being achievement, as individuals may not always pursue their well-being with that freedom.

Effective and Direct Freedom

As far as the process aspect of freedom is concerned, Sen makes an interesting and important distinction between 'effective freedom' and 'freedom as control'. Many of our freedoms may be enormously enhanced as a result of public policy, enabling us to pursue our objectives and achieve well-being without much exercise of active choice by ourselves. Public action should not only be concerned with an equitable enhancement of individual capabilities, but also with the 'efficient' enhancement of aggregate capabilities and freedoms, which have the effect of enhancing the effective freedoms of the population at large. For instance, the State undertakes numerous public health measures that enhance our freedoms to lead a healthy life collectively as well as individually, without us being involved in those measures or having direct control over our abilities or achievements to lead such a life. The fact that we can have a malaria-free life due to public health measures does not in any way compromise our capability to achieve a malaria-free life. In fact, given the complex nature of modern society, it is difficult to have a system in which we have direct control over every aspect of our lives. Our 'realized agency success' (based on 'effective freedoms' we enjoy, irrespective of our actual control over them) may not necessarily involve our 'instrumental agency success' (based on our participation or 'freedom as control' in our achievements). The latter is a 'seriously limited' view of freedom, which drastically reduces 'the scope and force of that great idea'. He argues that when Isaiah Berlin talked of 'a man's, or a people's, liberty to choose to live as they desire', the reference was not to their control over the mechanisms that afford them such a liberty, but their ability to make a choice of their living as they desire (Sen 1993, 1995a). Effective freedoms are especially relevant in the case of those who are not capable of exercising active choice for the achievement of their well-being, like small children particularly, the physically and mentally disabled, and others. In fact, one could argue that the lesser there is scope for direct choice and control over achievements or well-being, the greater the public responsibility to enhance the effective freedoms of concerned individuals. At the same time, it is important to highlight that, apart from our achievements, active choice contributes directly to our well-being when we have the capability to exercise such choice. We would take up this issue further a bit later.

Capabilities and Functionings

The capability approach generally concentrates on freedoms to achieve, but seems concerned with well-being freedoms and achievements in particular. The 'capability set' is a collection of alternative combinations of 'doings and beings' ('functionings'), from which a person can choose one combination that he has reason to value. It is not simply a set of any combinations from which a person *has* to choose, but one that is of value to him in view of his objectives and ends, so that it represents his 'real' opportunities. The metric of justice has to be sensitive not only to pervasive diversity in terms of internal characteristics and external circumstances of concerned individuals, but also to their diversity in terms of their ends and objectives they have reason to value (Sen 1995a). Achieved functionings—ranging from such elementary ones as being able to avoid premature mortality and being adequately nourished, to complex ones such as being able to achieve self-respect or to participate in the life of the community[14]—constitute well-being, and the capability to achieve them constitutes well-being freedom. It is important to note that a richer assessment of well-being and capabilities should *ideally* take into account the 'combination' of functionings that a person is able to manage, and not just a single functioning, since there might be trade-offs in their achievement. For instance, in order to avoid premature mortality, people may get indebted—healthcare is said to be the biggest cause of indebtedness in India[15]—or be forced to give up the pursuit of other important functionings because of lack of sufficient resources or other factors, and therefore the need to look at the entire set of functionings that a person is able to achieve. Nevertheless, this is not a non-negotiable requirement, and the selection of particular freedoms or functionings would depend on the purpose of evaluation at hand. For instance, if we wish to compare the survival advantage of various social groups, we might consider their life expectancy or mortality rates, and possibly a few other related functionings, but may not be interested in the entire gamut of functionings that those groups are able to achieve.

Capability Metric of Justice

Our assessments of justice should primarily be based on our well-being freedoms, and not generally on agency freedoms, for a 'society might accept some responsibility for a person's well-being, especially when that is in some danger of being particularly low'. However, it may not have to take an equal interest in the expansion of our non-well-being, agency objectives as well. However, again, whether the broad agency

[14] The utilitarian metric might count as an important functioning without, however, occupying a central place in capability assessments (Sen 1995a). Not just the utilitarian mental metrics, Sen does not allow such a place to any subjective metric, be it 'self-reported morbidity' (2002c) or our 'sense of injustice' (2009).

[15] According to a KPMG-OPPI report (2016: 6), 'nearly 63 million people are in debt due to health expenditure'.

or the more particular well-being aspect is given prominence depends on the purpose of the evaluation at hand ('plurality of purposes'). In the assessment of justice itself, we would have to go beyond the opportunity aspect of freedom at some level, even if that is the most significant aspect, and look at the process aspect as well (without placing it at the centre of our assessment), along with what people are able to do and be, that is, their actual achievements and well-being (Sen 2009). Nevertheless, even in considering our well-being aspect, we have to take the agency aspect into consideration as the former forms part of the latter and other non-well-being, agency aspects could affect well-being aspects too. Thus, the informationally rich evaluative framework does remain relevant (Sen 1995a).

Capabilities or Functionings?

Although the capability approach advocates a plurality of focus, the central focal variable is the freedoms or capabilities enjoyed by individuals.[16] Sen presents a variety of justifications for it: First, despite the fact that functionings are constitutive of well-being, the exercise of active choice, wherever possible, also contributes directly to our well-being. And since the achieved combination of functionings is one among the various combinations of functionings possible to us in a capability set, focusing on freedoms does not result in any informational loss, rather enriches the informational bases of our assessment.[17] Second, as mentioned earlier, there are objectives other than personal well-being that we may want to pursue through the exercise of our freedoms or capabilities, and since society is largely obligated to enhance our freedoms to pursue our personal well-being, and not necessarily all our other agency freedoms, we should place

[16] Equality and justice have to be concerned not only with how various countries and groups are doing vis-à-vis each other, but eventually with how individuals within them are doing—there are serious intra-country/-group/ -household inequities to be tackled. We cannot stop at any of the aggregates, down to the household level.

[17] Sen (1995a) has made a distinction between 'selection view', which focuses on the particular selection made, and 'options view', which not only takes into account the actual selection, but the options available.

capabilities at the heart of our assessments (without, of course, excluding achievements or processes, since capability evaluations have to be done in a 'desegregated way' (Sen 1993)).[18] Third, there is the issue of individual responsibility in the case of those who are capable of exercising their freedoms, and we should therefore look at their freedoms, and not their actual achievements, as they may not exercise their freedoms responsibly. 'The state may have reason to offer a person adequate opportunities to overcome hunger, but not to insist that he must take up that offer and cease to be hungry' (Sen 1993). Well-being achievement cannot be forced. Fourth, although achievements in terms of functionings *may* be a good guide to our underlying freedoms, since we usually give priority to our well-being if we have real opportunities to do so, this may not always be the case because our advantage in terms of achievements may reflect our biological advantage, for instance, and not our actual freedoms or procedural fairness, as may happen in the case of women, scheduled tribes (STs), and Muslims (this will be illustrated in the next chapter based on group-based mortality differentials in India). Therefore, it is important to concentrate on capabilities, as well as consider whether procedural fairness is being observed, along with evaluating functionings.

Basic Capabilities?

Sen introduced the notion of 'basic capabilities' for the evaluation of inequalities in his 1979 Tanner Lecture, 'Equality of What?'. He went on

---

[18] Sen has criticized utilitarianism for its exclusive focus on achievements and considering freedoms to achieve as totally instrumental. He sees Rawls' and Dworkin's focus on social primary goods and resources as a serious challenge to the exclusivist consequentialism of utilitarianism, marking a shift toward the assessment of freedom in the 'evaluative exercise'. However, he thinks the shift has not been adequate enough since their approaches do not duly take into account the fact of pervasive human diversity and other relevant factors that problematize the direct 'conversion' of resources into freedoms, leading to significant variations in achievements. As such, even resourcist perspectives fail to take account of the 'extent' of freedoms which people can enjoy (Sen 1995a).

to develop the capability approach which he later used for the analysis of well-being, living standards, poverty, development, liberty, freedom, social ethics, gender bias, justice, and so on. Although he argued that the use of the capability approach cannot be restricted to assessments of basic capabilities,[19] he thinks it is possible to have 'a fair amount of agreement on the extreme urgency of a class of needs', and so 'particular moral and political importance may well be attached to fulfilling well-recognized, urgent claims'. The case for focusing on a set of centrally relevant functionings and corresponding capabilities is indeed strong while we are dealing with extreme human deprivations, as in many parts of the developing world (Sen 1993, 1995a). Although he has often talked about deprivations in terms of the basic capabilities, he has been hesitant either in drawing up or endorsing any list of 'central human capabilities' as universally applicable—unlike Nussbaum (1997), who has drawn up one such list, which, although always tentative, seems to play a role similar to that of Rawls' social primary goods.

Sen (1993: 47) accepts 'that this would indeed be a systematic way of eliminating the incompleteness of the capability approach' and certainly has 'no great objection to anyone going on that route'. However, he does raise a number of objections against such an approach. One, he thinks that 'the use of the capability approach as such does not require taking that route, and the deliberate incompleteness of the capability approach permits other routes to be taken which also have some plausibility'. As such, he is not ready to accept it 'as the *only* route on which to travel', insisting on preserving the generality of the capability approach, as against making it 'a complete evaluative blueprint'. Two, from his perspective, 'this view of human nature (with a unique list of functionings for a good human life) may be tremendously overspecified', and might not resonate well with the pervasive diversity of human circumstances (internal and external) and choices. Three, he is worried about 'the nature and importance of the type of objectivity involved' (Sen 1993: 47). One could also add that a particular list includes certain things and also, by virtue of that, excludes others, things that may be quite important for many people who might not have been included in the process of developing that particular list. Such objections could be

[19] He did not identify 'certain capabilities as "basic" and others as not so' after the initial use of the term (Sen 1979, 1983).

raised regarding the erstwhile Millennium Development Goals (MDGs) and the present Sustainable Development Goal (SDGs), with both sets of goals strongly oriented towards specific outcomes rather than freedoms.

The Measurement of Justice

It is important to discuss some of the relevant issues pertaining to the measurement of justice within the capability framework.

One, justice is to be *eventually* measured at the individual, not the social, level, although our choice will be governed by the evaluative purpose on hand. However, ultimately, based on the availability of relevant data, the focus should ideally be on how individuals within and across groups are doing. Our individual capabilities are, in many instances, influenced by what has been termed 'collective capabilities' (Deneulin 2008). It is possible that one is not able to adequately understand the capability-deprivations of individuals within the groups without appreciating the collective capability-deprivations that the group faces at the aggregate level. However, that would be a part of our empirical concern, but does not necessarily have to be so at a normative level. Measuring capabilities at the level of the groups could potentially mask serious intra-group deprivations. For example, as Sen has pointed out, the wealth status of a household does not tell us about the actual distribution of resources within the family, and it is quite possible that females and others get discriminated at this and other levels. Thus, not only should we look beyond resources, but beyond all sorts of aggregates, including the family, as far as equality and justice are concerned. Justice, in Sen's framework, appears to demand nothing less than disaggregation to the ultimate level, and does not stop until it reaches the individual, because it is possible that 'social' justice is enhanced, even when 'individual' justice is not. Scheduled castes (SCs) in the north-Indian state of Uttar Pradesh, for instance, are doing better now than they were before, but are all their sub-castes (there were 66 in the state as on 26 October 2017, according to India's Union Ministry of Social Justice and Empowerment) and all individuals within those sub-castes doing better? We would get a very different assessment based on this perspective. Responding to Evans's (2002) use of the term as a sociological critique of Sen's individualistic focus,

Sen (2002a: 85) does talk of 'collective capabilities', but argues that a better description is *socially dependent individual capabilities* (emphasis as per original). However, this does not mean that an assessment of collective capabilities is unimportant; it is extremely important, especially in cases of entrenched forms of 'social' injustice. At the same time, we need to look at the individual impact of social justice or injustice, since neither does everyone benefit equally from positive measures, nor is everybody equally affected by social evils, corruption, governmental inefficiency, and so on. The poor and the weak, for instance, usually tend to benefit less and suffer more. One could also argue that in the assessments of *what has not been achieved*, we should look at the 'social' as well as other dimensions, including the individual; but when it comes to the final assessment of *what has been achieved*, the ultimate focus should be on the individual.

Second, Sen argues that concepts like well-being and inequality (and one could add justice, freedom, and capability here) are 'broad and partly opaque', and 'may have enough ambiguity and fuzziness to make it a mistake to look for a complete ordering of either' in terms of inter-personal comparisons and evaluations.[20] However, rather than staying totally silent until we have absolute clarity, we can undertake their evaluations based on those aspects on which we can obtain even partial rankings in an unambiguous manner (Sen 1995a). Another issue is the lack of relevant data that can capture these concepts adequately. Nevertheless, despite the 'vagueness of the underlying concepts' and 'the gaps in the relevant data', we need to be sure,

---

[20] It is interesting to note the following from Sen (2006a: 45–6): 'If we want a properly satisfactory measure of inequality or poverty, we cannot define it over the income space alone, and have to supplement the income data by information about social relations between people.... Economic data cannot be interpreted without the necessary sociological understanding', and we still have 'a long way to go still to make adequate social sense of economic measures.' However, though the capability approach does not, at least in principle, rule out the use of qualitative methods in the understanding or measurement of inequality, poverty, injustice, and so on, Sen has shown a strong preference for hard data based on quantitative methods and measures, which seems more reliable to him. However, Sen's complex and multi-disciplinary approach to the understanding of inequality—or poverty and development more generally—is worthwhile.

in principle, how the analysis would have been done if it was possible to get rid of these ambiguities and non-availability of relevant data. This does not imply that we should not seek conceptual clarity since 'informational lacuna or complexity of concepts need not serve as an excuse for tolerating avoidable conceptual murkiness'. Difficulties in observing the utilitarian metric did not prevent it from becoming the dominant paradigm in moral philosophy and welfare economics for a very long time (Sen 2000b).

Nevertheless, it needs to be pointed out that there are certain basic aspects of these concepts which are not that difficult to capture unambiguously—and for which data is also available—for us to undertake inter-personal comparisons. In addition, some of these are used as summary measures of our well-being. The capability to avoid premature mortality is one of the most fundamental.

Nothing matters unless we are alive, and hence the capability to survive and avoid premature mortality is indisputably the most basic human capability, and there is thus a special practical case for focusing on it in our assessment of justice, equality, well-being, and capabilities. And, as Sen argues, when we evaluate inequalities in this and other such basic capabilities, 'we are not merely examining differences in well-being, but also in the basic freedoms that we value and cherish'—they 'tell us a great deal about the presence or absence of certain central basic *freedoms*' and 'given the motivation underlying the analysis of inequality, it is important not to miss this momentous perspective'. It is crucial to emphasize that 'even simple observations of realized states may have direct relevance to the analysis of freedoms enjoyed' (Sen 1995a). As such, child survival could well be regarded as an indicator of direct assessment of justice.

Coming to premature mortality as an indicator of the well-being of the population, Sen argues that it has dual relevance—it not only tells us about death, but also provides signals of illness, sufferings, and miseries in concerned populations. He points to a number of potential benefits of focusing on it: One, it tells us about something which is of fundamental intrinsic relevance, and not of derivative instrumental value as incomes. Two, the freedoms and capabilities that we value 'are contingent on our being alive'. Three, not only this, mortality data tells us a lot about our other capabilities and functionings. 'There might often be relatively limited tension between the virtue of raising life expectancy and many other elementary accomplishments central to the process of development', and mortality data, thus, 'can, to some extent, serve as a proxy for associated failures and achievements to which we may attach importance'. Four, data on mortality is usually more readily available than on many other such vital capabilities. Five, gender bias, which is 'very hard to identify, since many of the discriminations are subtle and covert, and lie within the core of intimate family behaviour', could be well-reflected in gender-based mortality differentials as well as in sex ratio. Mortality differentials provide an entry into racial and other such inequalities which could be seriously missed if our 'analysis were to be confined only to traditional economic variables' such as incomes (Sen 1998). However, it is important to note that mortality differentials may not always reveal underlying inequities, as the next chapter on child survival amply demonstrates— marginalized groups such as STs and Muslims actually have had an advantage in child survival.

Consistent with his insistence on objectively measurable and monitorable indicators, Sen has argued that while mortality may be quite a reliable indicator of our well-being, 'self-reported morbidity' may not be. Taking Kerala as an example, he asks whether its high morbidity rates provide a really good indication of its level of health or well-being, and whether Keralites are worse off vis-à-vis their counterparts in Bihar, Uttar Pradesh, and Madhya Pradesh, who have much lower morbidity rates but much higher mortality rates. To him, morbidity data tends to suffer from 'major biases'. Our understanding of morbidity and illness is dependent on our medical knowledge as well as on the kind of healthcare we are used to receiving. When people have a good deal of health awareness and care, they have a heightened sense of health and illnesses, and vice versa. It is, thus, not surprising that self-reported morbidity rates are higher in the US than in Kerala. He raised the problem of 'positional objectivity' and 'observational biases' in morbidity-reporting, that is, morbidity seen from a different position or perspective—for instance, through a clinical lens—may yield a very different reading (Sen 1995c). Nevertheless, he feels that, generally, we can avoid 'the narrowness and limitation of choosing *either* the internal *or* the external perspective'—that is, of self-reported (internal) and clinically-proven (external) morbidity—or the 'self-inflicted injury of methodological narrowness and dogmatism', by committing to an 'open-minded epistemology', which does not insist on choosing one and rejecting the other (Sen 2006b; emphases as per original). For him, 'the point at issue is not that of *ignoring* the self-perception of illness', but interpreting and enriching it through mortality data (Sen 1998; emphasis as per original). Not just a plurality of focal variables and purposes, but of methods too.

Children and the Capability Approach

Although the capability approach 'has not yet adequately engaged with children's issues' (Biggeri, Ballet, and Comim 2011), it appears more suited than other metrics for the analysis and comparisons of children's advantage. However, it still needs to be considered whether in the case of small children, with whom we are concerned—do we rather look at their functionings as capabilities and freedoms *might* not mean much for them? Why is it important to take into account freedom to achieve at the level of basic capabilities in the case of children as well as generally when what really matters at that level is basic human survival, nutrition, and so on? It is relatively easier to appreciate why freedoms are important at higher levels of functioning. It also gives rise to the question—how much does capability-enhancement really matter when there is a crisis and children are dying in millions every year?

If we insist on making assessments of child survival in the capability space, should we focus directly on children's capability to survive or their parent's capabilities to provide conditions for their survival? If children are dependent on their parents, and the latter are responsible for their well-being, a responsibility which they are expected to fulfil with the best that they can, and small children in any case lack agency or freedom of their own, or the knowledge of what is good and bad for them, should we not just focus on their parent's capabilities who promote their survival? As far as the spirit of capability approach is concerned, we should rather focus on children's capabilities directly (direct assessment) as parents' capabilities may not *convert* straightforwardly into their children's capabilities.

This also links up to the issue as to who all is responsible for children's survival and well-being? In situations when parents are not taking care of their children well—or do not have the capability of doing so—should the State intervene and take care of children?[21] Sex-selective abortion is illegal in countries like India, so the State does intervene to ensure child survival at the pre-natal level. Empirical evidence suggests that we cannot always take the family to be a benign and egalitarian unit in all cases—especially females, including children—and thus, in the final analysis, the capability of the individual concerned (that is, of children directly) should be the focus of our assessment. Nevertheless, it needs to be taken into account that the younger the child, the more dependant it is on its parents—access to prenatal care at the biomedical level as well as parental economic and educational status are significant contributors to early child survival. So, the well-being of parents, especially the mother, cannot be completely ignored, even if we are concerned with justice for children. This is where lies a major challenge for all those who argue for focusing on individuals in assessments of justice—in the case of child survival, focus cannot only be on the child itself, but on its mother in particular, and the household more generally, although the ultimate focus would be on the child itself. Child survival is one sphere in which a 'non-individual' approach to justice is essential.

Conceptual Assessment of the Capability Approach

This section undertakes a general and specific (to the issue of child survival) assessment of Sen's approach as discussed above at a conceptual level. It undertakes a contextual assessment based on child mortality and access to determinants of child survival among selected Indian groups. However, the criticisms raised here do not mean that Sen's approach is irrelevant from our perspective—they are meant to highlight areas of weakness in which the capability approach can be refined further as far as justice for children is concerned.

---

[21] For Sen (2008b: 276), 'the social commitment' to freedoms does not have to 'operate only through the state, but must also involve other institutions: political and social organizations, community-based arrangements, non-governmental agencies of various kinds, the media and other means of public understanding and communication, and the institutions that allow the functioning of markets and contractual relations'.

Equality or Efficiency?

For Sen (1995a: 15), 'equality would typically be one consideration among many', while 'a lexicographic priority of equality over aggregative considerations' is 'possibly over-strong'. In contrast, Rawls started out *A Theory of Justice* with an 'intuitive conviction' regarding the primacy of justice: 'justice is the first virtue of social institutions', and 'each person possesses an inviolability founded on justice that even the welfare of society as a whole cannot override' (Rawls 1971: 3–4)—whose 'general tendency' he could assess and support by means of his theory of 'justice as fairness' (1971: 586). Furthermore, the first part of his 'Difference Principle' demands that 'social and economic inequalities are to be arranged so that they are both ... to the greatest benefit of the least advantaged' (1971: 83). Though these demands may seem too extreme, inflexible, or unifocal, we cannot avoid systematically dealing with the issue of priority at some level, even if in a dramatically watered-down style or with contextual riders. Sen's approach in this case seems congruent with his overall style of non-specific inclusivity. He seems to be wanting to include too much and specifying too little, which can be particularly challenging from a policy perspective. In contrast, both Rawls and Nozick, for instance, seem to come out clearly and strongly in support of their focus and central focal variables. Sen sounds conceptually what anthropologists, for instance, tend to sound empirically—things are complex and it is difficult to come up with explicit solutions.

Equality of What, Exactly?

Sen does not appear to have dealt with the issue of equalisandum in his framework with much clarity, to say the least. First, he has intensively and extensively argued in favour of focusing on the space of capabilities in a way that one gets an impression that the capability approach, as the name also suggests, is about the equality of capabilities or freedoms, which, as we saw above, he did argue for in so many words, in a number of places, although he refused to do so in *The Idea of Justice* (Sen 2009). The clarifications that he has given in the latter work for not supporting 'equality *of* capability' do not come out prominently in his previous works.

Second, he has argued against a unifocal approach (in the context of equality in general, as well as of health equity in particular), and in favour of focal plurality or 'multiple dimensions in which equality matters' (Sen 2009). However, while he talks about trade-offs between the various dimensions (2009: 295), that pervasive human diversity can make equality in different spaces 'non-congruent—indeed, frequently far apart' (Sen 1995a), he does not specify which dimension within his multifocal variable would have priority. Although one might assume that the dimension of capability and freedom would have priority—at least in the case of adults capable of choice, an assumption which could be supported by some of his writings—it does not actually come out very clearly if we look at some of his major writings as a whole. Particularly when he brings other equity concerns (processes, achievements) into discussion, his style tends to be inclusivist, non-committal, unwilling to spell out a clear-cut priority even in specific contextual cases, let alone at a general or conceptual level (with contextual riders).

For example, while talking about women's biological advantage in survival, Sen (2002b: 24) says that 'the process aspect of justice and equity demand some attention, without necessarily occupying the centre of the stage'. Elsewhere (2009: 296), he argues that 'it is not unreasonable to claim that, in cases of this kind, demands of equity in the process aspect of freedom could sensibly override any single-minded concentration on the opportunity aspect of freedom, including prioritizing equality in life expectancy'. In the former, it seems he recognizes the problem that the issue of women's biological advantage poses to his concentration on the space of capabilities and functionings, and responds with 'some attention' to the demands of procedural fairness. In the latter, he appears willing to allow process equity to even 'sensibly override' his strong primordial focus on capabilities and functionings, even in the context of such an elementary functioning as survival and life expectancy. This seems to emerge from Sen's hesitation in clearly specifying the conceptual and contextual priority which should be attached to the constituents of his multifocal variable. In fact, in his initial writings, procedural fairness was not as prominently discussed or defended as were capabilities and functionings. In fact, at one place, he even argued that 'these variables [relating to the *means* of capabilities or functionings] are not part of the evaluative space, though they can indirectly influence the evaluation through their effects on variables included in that space' (Sen 1993). In later works (Sen 2006b: 24; 2009: 296), he claimed that 'it would be morally unacceptable to suggest that women should receive worse health care than men' and 'giving women less medical attention than men for the same health problems would flagrantly violate a significant requirement of process equity'.

It also seems problematic from an empirical perspective to simply assume that, 'given similar health care and other forms of attention, women tend to have a lower mortality rate than men do at nearly all age groups' (Sen 1998). Sen does not provide any proof of this, and goes on to make claims of procedural justice in favour of women based on their assumed biological universal advantage, without considering the possibility of cultural and other differentiations. It may be possible that in some cultures or countries, women possess a genetic predisposition, for instance, that enables them to live longer than women in other cultures or countries.

One could argue that our metrics of justice should be sensitive to what is possible—and this especially holds true in the case of Sen, who has argued for focusing on removal of manifest and redressable injustices or on unambiguous inequities, rather than on 'perfect justice'—and the comments below, even if not directly related to the discussion of the metric of justice, are relevant in terms of their consequences for the consideration of a realistic choice of space. Following are certain comments which directly or indirectly relate to Sen's metric.

1. Continuing with the issue of women, Sen only refers to their biological advantage while talking of procedural fairness. What about individuals or certain other social or cultural or genetic groups who could be biologically advantaged? Or, in general, all those who might need lesser resources to develop required capabilities? Should they get less healthcare and other benefits just because they are better endowed? Are we not obliged to observe process equity in all such cases, or is this provision only for women? If process equity is for all, where is the rationale for focusing on capabilities based on human diversity? Should female advantage not be seen as one of the dimensions of that diversity (there could be other axes of human diversity)? In addition, if you talk about individual assessment at the end of the day, why particularly invoke only one social category (gender) and not

others? Second, from Sen's own logic, equality in one space tends to clash with equality in other spaces; hence his question, *equality of what?* How, then, do we take into account equity in both procedural as well as opportunity dimensions at the same time? Even if it is possible, we should specify the space in which equity has priority, even if not in an absolutist or exclusivist sense.

2. Linked to this is the issue of discrimination, an important aspect which justice is supposed to address, irrespective of material consequences. Despite his persistent exhortation to go beyond a resourcist approach, Sen himself seems to give priority to material well-being even when he talks about freedoms—mostly with reference to it—and has not really discussed the challenge of discrimination per se as far as justice is concerned. While other political philosophers could also be accused of this omission, those who focus on procedural fairness are less vulnerable to this sort of accusation. Sen too argues in favour of taking it into consideration, but (*a*) it is not as pronounced; and (*b*) he still does not specifically discuss the challenge of discrimination, although he is concerned with its consequences, at the individual level. Like several public health evils, discrimination is a social evil which must be addressed, first and foremost, at a societal level. It is not a secondary concern which can be subsumed under either the comprehensive umbrella of Rawls' social primary goods or Sen's capabilities. There has to be an explicit consideration in our discussions of justice to deal with it. Moreover, it is not a higher order concern, which can be considered after deprivations of basic capabilities or manifest injustices have been addressed—these things often come about directly as a result of discrimination. Nevertheless, let us also quote him in his own defense (Sen 2006a: 45), 'if we want a properly satisfactory measure of inequality or poverty, we cannot define it over the income space alone, and have to supplement the income data by information about social relations.... Economic data cannot be interpreted without the necessary sociological understanding.' This remark can also be invoked later to argue against not focusing on the pursuit of social justice on such metrics as caste, race, and so on. Nevertheless, as reflected by the earlier discussion, Sen still sees the economic (material) dimension as primary and 'information about social relations' as supplemental.

3. Sen does not seem to have talked about the role of luck in the formation of capabilities—which he has rarely discussed—or in achieving functionings based on one's capabilities, and it is possible that no matter how much support we have or how much capable we are, some of us may not be able to develop certain capabilities or achieve some functionings (which could also be due to our lack of knowledge about *each* determinant of capabilities or achievements). There is a group of prominent political philosophers referred to as 'luck egalitarians' who argue that justice should prioritize a focus on the condition of those affected by simple bad luck—Ronald Dworkin, G.A. Cohen, John Roemer, Thomas Nagel, and Richard Arneson being a few theorists in this broad and diverse strand of thought. Sen has discussed their work in several places, but has not dealt with the issue of luck prominently. In the Indian context, it is particularly relevant since a dominant view is that the disadvantaged people are suffering from bad luck due to their bad actions (*karma*) in their previous life. Whether the roots of what we refer to as 'bad luck' are otherworldly or social, it has to part of our public policy on justice. Having said that, one could argue that luck could be subsumed under the diversity of human diversity that Sen talked about. However, some of the forms that this 'black box' of inexplicable realities could assume may make equity in processes or capabilities quite difficult, and therefore deserves to be treated explicitly. And then we also have a major strand of justice literature dealing with this issue.

4. Since luck and State capability to prevent premature mortality are contextual, we would need specific local accounts that separate misfortune (which cannot be prevented) from injustice (which can be prevented), and, therefore, what may be an injustice in a particular context may not necessarily be so in another context. Knowledge of differential capabilities of States in enhancing the capabilities of citizens would also be relevant in making such distinctions. Sen does not seem to have dealt with such issues. Part of the evaluation should also be differential global or local complexities that various States have to deal with. Sen is, therefore, justified in pointing to the relevance of the demands of efficiency with equality. All sources of human diversity are not amenable to public or private action—there is enormous diversity

of State capacities too—and, thus, it may never be possible to have equality of capabilities—Sen is, therefore, justified in being hesitant about arguing for equality of capabilities unifocally.

5. The issue of State or individual responsibility in the formation of capabilities or achievements has not been adequately discussed in Sen's work, a view supported by Roemer (1996), and unless we fix responsibility, we can neither identify nor address injustice, as discussed in the previous chapter. Since we cannot hold non-governmental organizations responsible in this regard due to the voluntary nature of their work, does ultimate responsibility lie on the State? Sen has defined 'public action' as not just action by the State, but the entire array of stakeholders. However, how it works in the context of 'responsibility', is one of the most central notions in discussions of justice and injustice. Who is responsible for committing injustices and who is responsible for addressing those injustices?

6. Finally, and probably most importantly, as far as the politics of social justice in India and the US is concerned, Sen has confined himself to metrics as proposed in the political philosophical litera-ture and has not gone on to assess those based on which affirma-tive action policies have been made in two of the world's largest democracies, where there has been a great deal of contention on the issue and has affected much of their politics. No other major political philosopher, too, appears to have done so, but given Sen's focus on actual and redressable injustices, one could at least expect it from him. There seems to be a fundamental conceptual impli-cation too of this omission. Confined to theoretical literature, he focused the major part of his energies on criticizing the resourcist/ utilitarian approaches to justice and arguing that we need to go beyond resources as there is enormous human diversity and these metrics do not tell us about our capabilities to achieve valuable functionings. What about the practice of social justice based on caste or race? Can we make a similar set of arguments about going beyond these traditional axes of injustice—given pervasive human diversity and their failure to explain or address the injustice faced by individuals within and across castes and races? In comparison to the pursuit of social justice based on caste or race—or, for that matter, other background variables such as gender, religion, and

so on—a resourcist approach actually appears better since we are actually focusing on the condition of individuals—or households, the level at which poverty is considered in India policy. Clearly, a capability focus is even better, but if we are criticizing other dominant approaches, we need to put the spotlight at least as much on caste, race, and other background variables as much as resources, if we are concerned with practical policy in at least two nations with major programs to address historical injustices. In the name of gender justice, too, in India, it is usually the privileged women who benefit, while the fortunes of the disadvantaged ones does not seem to change much. If resources do not always reflect our capabilities, privileged social background does not as well, always. Eventually, we need to move on and consider the capabilities of individuals.

Functionings as Indicators of Freedom

Our freedoms lie between inputs (resources, rights, and so on) and outputs (functionings), and the problem of 'conversion' can apply at both levels (of inputs into freedoms, of freedoms into outputs)—due to the fact of pervasive human diversity at the first level, and due to individual responsibility and non-well-being agency pursuits at the second level. But while Sen takes the advocates of procedural fairness to task for focusing on resources or rights, criticizing their metrics of being inadequate in telling us about the extents of freedoms we enjoy, he makes rationalistic assumptions on behalf of human actors at the second level and sees little problem in taking achievements as a guide (though not completely reliable) to our freedoms. Consider this from him, for example: 'in most situations, health achievement tends to be a good guide to the underlying capabilities, since we tend to give priority to good health when we have the real opportunity to choose' (Sen 2006b). He also talks of 'counterfactual choices (what we *would* choose)', and argues that in some cases, it is easy to guess our counterfactual choices, and in those, 'realized states may have direct relevance to the analysis of freedoms enjoyed' (Sen 1995a). He often uses the term 'reason to value'—people may not always have a reason to value something, they may just value it out of an idiosyncrasy—not a far-fetched thought, especially in a world and era where Donald Trump could become the president of the world's biggest democracy and economy. The pervasive fact of human diversity in terms of choices and ends perhaps applies here as in other realms, and it is not clear to what extent can we make assumptions of rational, counterfactual choices on behalf of human actors. On the other hand, he criticized Rawls for assuming selfless rationality on behalf of participants in the 'original position' behind 'a veil of ignorance'. This argument, however, does not militate against focusing on functionings since they are of intrinsic value, while inputs are not. Second, this argument does not also apply so much in evaluations of justice with reference to those incapable of responsibility or choice—small children and some categories of disabled people, in whose cases, 'realized states' could be a highly, though not a completely, reliable guide to the 'effective freedoms' they possess.

Despite these criticisms, the complexity that Sen has brought to the discussion on metrics of justice through his advocacy for a multifocal variable is appreciable and makes his approach, in an overall sense, much more relevant to the kind of complex context that we have in a country like India. As indicated at the beginning of the introduction, simple approaches to justice have created problems in India and elsewhere and we, therefore, need more complex approaches to justice to prevent the slide towards fragility, both as a result of the lack and backlash against the prevalent practices of social justice. However, we would need to make several conceptual and contextual adjustments to his approach to make it meaningful for our purpose in this book. That should not be a problem as 'the strength of Sen's vision consists of its openness' (Alexander 2010: 77).

References

Alexander, John M. 2010. *Capabilities and Social Justice. The Political Philosophy of Amartya Sen and Martha Nussbaum*. Farnham: Ashgate.

Anand, Sudhir, Fabienne Peter, and Amartya Sen, eds. 2006. *Public Health, Ethics and Equity*. Oxford: Oxford University Press.

Aristotle. 1996. *The Nicomachean Ethics*. Edited and translated by Harris Rackham. Hertfordshire: Wordsworth.

Basu, Kaushik, and Ravi Kanbur, eds. 2009. *Arguments for a Better World: Essays in Honor of Amartya Sen. Vol. 1: Ethics, Welfare, and Measurement*. New York: Oxford University Press.

Biggeri, Mario, Jérôme Ballet, and Flavio Comim, eds. 2011. *Children and the Capability Approach*. Houndmills, Basingstoke, Hampshire, New York: Palgrave Macmillan.

Deneulin, Séverine. 2008. 'Beyond Individual Freedom and Agency: Structures of Living together in Sen's Capability Approach to Development'. In *The Capability Approach: Concepts, Measures and Applications*, edited by Flavio Comim, Mozaffar Qizilbash, and Sabina Alkire, 105–24. Cambridge: Cambridge University Press.

Evans, Peter. 2002. 'Collective Capabilities, Culture, and Amartya Sen's Development as Freedom: Symposium on "Development as Freedom" by Amartya Sen'. *Studies in Comparative International Development* 37 (2): 54–60.

KPMG and OPPI. 2016. 'Report on healthcare access initiatives'. https://home. kpmg.com/in/en/home/insights/2016/08/report-on-healthcare-access-initiatives.html (accessed 28 July 2018).

Marx, Karl, and Friedrich Engels. 1998. *The German Ideology. Including 'Theses on Feuerbach' and 'Introduction to the Critique of Political Economy'*. New York: Prometheus Books.

Nozick, Robert. 1974. *Anarchy, State, and Utopia*. Oxford and Cambridge, MA: Blackwell.

Nussbaum, Martha. 1987. *Nature, Function, and Capability: Aristotle on Political Distribution*. World Institute for Development Economics Research of the United Nations University.

———. 1997. 'Capabilities and human rights'. *Fordham Law Review*, 66 (2): 273–300.

Rawls, John. 1971. *A Theory of Justice*. Cambridge, MA: The Belknap Press of Harvard University Press.

Roemer, John. 1996. *Theories of Distributive Justice*. Cambridge, MA: Harvard University Press.

Sen, Amartya. 1979. *Equality of What?* The Tanner Lecture on Human Values. Stanford: Stanford University.

———. 1983. 'Poor, Relatively Speaking'. *Oxford Economic Papers* 35 (2): 153–69.

———. 1985. *Commodities and Capabilities*. Amsterdam, North-Holland: Elsevier Science.

———. 1988. 'Freedom of Choice: Concept and Content'. *European Economic Review* 32 (2–3): 269–94.

———. 1993. 'Capability and Well-being'. In *The Quality of Life*, edited by Martha Nussbaum and Amartya Sen. Oxford: Clarendon Press.

———. 1995a. *Inequality Reexamined*. New York: Russell Sage Foundation; Cambridge, MA: Harvard University Press.

————. 1995b. 'Gender Inequality and Theories of Justice'. In *Women, Culture and Development: A Study of Human Capabilities*, edited by Martha Nussbaum and Jonathan Glover, 259–74. Oxford: Clarendon Press.

————. 1995c. *Health, Inequality and Welfare Economics*. Thiruvananthapuram: Center for Development Studies.

————. 1998. 'Mortality as an Indicator of Economic Success and Failure'. *The Economic Journal* 108 (446): 1–25.

————. 2000a. *Development as Freedom*. New York: Anchor Books.

————. 2000b. 'Social Justice and the Distribution of Income'. In *Handbook of Income Distribution: Volume 1*, edited by Anthony B. Atkinson and François Bourguignon, 59–85. Amsterdam and Oxford, North-Holland: Elsevier Science.

————. 2002a. 'Response to Commentaries: Symposium on Development as Freedom by Amartya Sen'. *Studies in Comparative International Development* 37 (2): 78–86.

————. 2002b. 'Why Health Equity?' *Health Economics* 11: 659–66.

————. 2002c. 'Health: Perception versus Observation'. *British Medical Journal* 324 (7342): 860–1.

————. 2003. 'Development as Capability Expansion'. In *Readings in Human Development: Concepts, Measures and Policies for a Development Paradigm*, edited by Sakiko Fukuda-Parr and A.K. Shiva Kumar. New Delhi and New York: Oxford University Press.

————. 2004. *On Ethics and Economics*. Oxford: Blackwell.

————. 2006a. 'Conceptualizing and Measuring Poverty'. In *Poverty and Inequality*, edited by David Grusky and Ravi Kanbur, 30–46. Stanford: Stanford University Press.

————. 2006b. 'Health Achievement and Equity: External and Internal Perspectives'. In *Public Health, Ethics and Equity*, edited by Sudhir Anand, Fabienne Peter, and Amartya Sen, 263–8. Oxford: Oxford University Press.

————. 2008a. 'The Economics of Happiness and Capability'. In *Capabilities & Happiness*, edited by Luigino Bruni, Flavio Comim, and Maurizio Pugno, 16–27. New York: Oxford University Press.

————. 2008b. 'Individual Freedom as a Social Commitment'. In *Daily Struggles: The Deepening Racialization and Feminization of Poverty in Canada*, edited by Maria A. Wallis and Siu-Ming Kwok, 275–87. Toronto: Canadian Scholars' Press.

————. 2009. *The Idea of Justice*. Cambridge, MA: The Belknap Press of Harvard University Press.

3

The Prospects of Survival

Child survival in India is unjust, first and foremost, at the systemic level, which is reflected in the country's poor aggregative performance over the decades. The persistent, systemic neglect of child survival in Indian policy architecture—the narrow focus on biomedical Reproductive and Child Health (RCH) notwithstanding— has meant that even otherwise well-off groups have not done so well. We do not have to go too far to appreciate the impact of such systemic neglect or even the performance of our RCH programme. In neighbouring Maldives, those with no or primary education had a lower U5MR (34) in 2009 than those with secondary or higher education in India (36) in 2015–16, while those in the lowest wealth index in the former had a U5MR (28) which was slightly worse than those in the highest wealth index in the latter (25), as per their respective Demographic and Health Surveys (DHS). Likewise, the percentage of under-five children severely stunted (below the –3 standard deviation of height for age according to WHO) among those in the lowest wealth index in Maldives was slightly less (7.4) than those among the highest wealth index in India (7.8) in 2015–16. The figures for under-five children severely wasted (below the –3 standard deviation of weight for height according to WHO) were 2.8 and 6.5 respectively.[1] Those who are used

---

[1] These figures were taken from STATcompiler on the DHS website https://www.statcompiler.com/en/ (accessed on 5 August 2018). Rates are for ten years preceding the survey.

to living in denial of such realities—and there is no dearth of them in the country—would immediately jump up to argue that Maldives is not comparable vis-à-vis our population size, diversity and democracy, and it is, thus, easy for them to achieve such outcomes easily. One can put forth many examples to demonstrate a similar trend, but let us leave at that—the Indian government elite is committed to, always ready to justify, systemic failures and injustices, shoot down arguments for systemic change and preserve the status quo.

Beyond them, the literature on the political economy of health as well as proponents of global justice could argue that the capability of the Indian State to address health challenges such as child mortality has remained limited due to given international order, power structures and relations, and we should, therefore, blame the latter for the so-called systemic neglect by the former. My own contention is that national political will can overcome the impact of global injustice, even when it is actually there—which one could doubt in the case of India, given that it has been a major global power to reckon with, for some decades at least—substantially, if not completely. Let us take the case of Iran and Cuba, two countries that have faced international sanctions led by the US for a very long time. Iran was not only one of the best performers on MDG 4, which is related to child survival, but is among the top 10 performing countries vis-à-vis the SDGs in general. Cuba, on the other hand, has had better child and general health indicators than the US itself, despite spending way much less on healthcare per capita. Not just vis-à-vis Cuba, the US has been the world's largest spender on healthcare, with its health outcomes incommensurate with its spending level—another case demonstrating why a resourcist approach to health is deficient. Without international sanctions, both these countries could have done much better, and so there is definitely a case for focusing on global injustice as well. As far as political will is concerned, we have the example of Nepal and Bangladesh in our own neighbourhood, who are doing much better than India on child mortality despite much fewer resources. But again, none of them is comparable to India! We also discuss China's case, which although more populous than India, lacks its diversity and democracy! This narrative only strengthens our argument of persistent, systemic neglect and injustice that has kept India lagging on child survival and other indicators of growth and development, keeping it from realizing its capabilities/potential.

Overlooking the aggregative, systemic challenge of child survival and focusing exclusively on inter-group/-individual inequalities would mean a narrow understanding and consideration of injustice. As such, we begin this chapter with a brief discussion of India's performance on child survival vis-à-vis the other top five contributing countries as far as the number of under-five deaths is concerned—*number*, since every child has a right to life, which the *rate* of under-five deaths does not quite capture—as well as the performance of Indian states, given that health is a state subject in India. We then discuss inter- and intra-group inequalities in child survival—after a brief justification as to why we are focusing on them, not inter-individual inequalities per se.

Inter-Country Comparisons

Under-Five Deaths

India has been the world's biggest contributor to all levels of child deaths[2] since 1953 (Table 3.1). Starting with 4.65 million under-five deaths a year, mortality decline in the initial three decades was slow, but gained momentum in 1986, four years before the MDG reference year (1990) and five years before market reforms were formally launched (1991). In fact, in China—the world's second largest contributor to under-five deaths until 1994—there was a mortality decline of 2.4 million in the decade before the market reforms of 1979, which were not only the most dramatic ever in the country, but in any country in human history in terms of the number of deaths. There was actually a substantial reversal in gains between 1983 and 1990 in China, but declines in the decade after were again quite dramatic. On the other hand, decline in India has always been incremental vis-à-vis China, with the country recording more than double the number of under-five deaths than

---

[2] Neonatal deaths refers to deaths within the first month of life, post-neonatal deaths to deaths between the first and twelfth months of life, infant deaths includes them both, while child deaths refer to deaths between the first and fifth years of life, and under-five deaths to all deaths from birth up to the age of five years.

TABLE 3.1 Levels of Child Mortality (Numbers) among Top Five Contributors to Global Under-Five Deaths (1990)

Country	1953	1969	1980	1990	2000	2010	2015	Decline (%), 1990–2015
			Number of Under-Five Deaths					
India	4,652,419	4,415,300	4,006,844	3,357,317	2,513,120	1,595,122	1,200,998	64
China		3,657,016	1,189,177	1,633,808	585,027	251,554	181,574	89
Nigeria		697,907	690,697	848,601	929,285	811,738	750,111	12
Pakistan	527,614	447,099	505,054	592,722	496,972	470,193	431,568	27
Bangladesh	542,941	651,347	688,845	527,587	316,983	157,890	119,326	77
			Number of Infant Deaths					
India	3,192,325	2,939,019	2,735,130	2,338,465	1,828,921	1,225,179	946,304	60
China		2,652,450	874,764	1,318,731	472,967	216,375	156,450	88
Nigeria		409,803	413,614	501,644	564,728	513,166	484,368	3
Pakistan	372,853	335,039	385,992	458,674	387,658	382,955	350,600	24
Bangladesh	354,766	437,419	471,016	363,463	231,531	123,231	97,478	73
			Infant Deaths as Percentage of Under-Five Deaths					
India	69	67	68	70	73	77	79	−13
China		73	74	81	81	86	86	−7
Nigeria		59	60	59	61	63	65	−9
Pakistan	71	75	76	77	78	81	81	−5
Bangladesh	65	67	68	69	73	78	82	−19

(Cont'd)

TABLE 3.1 (Cont'd)

Country	1953	1969	1980	1990	2000	2010	2015	Decline (%), 1990–2015
				Number of Neonatal Deaths				
India		1,755,942	1,743,574	1,537,008	1,253,657	871,304	695,852	55
China				928,027	331,419	131,241	93,435	90
Nigeria		162,335	176,042	200,678	243,837	241,117	240,106	−20
Pakistan		175,636	225,978	281,037	270,407	263,193	244,746	13
Bangladesh		281,077	311,876	233,880	154,428	91,438	74,378	68
				Neonatal Deaths as Percentage of Infant Deaths				
India		60	64	66	69	71	74	−12
China				70	70	61	60	15
Nigeria		40	43	40	43	47	50	−24
Pakistan		52	59	61	70	69	70	−14
Bangladesh		64	66	64	67	74	76	−19

Source: United Nations Inter-agency Group for Child Mortality database (IGME).

China at the beginning of the MDG period (1990) and more than six times by the end of it (2015).

Nevertheless, starting out with a much higher level, India's contribution to global under-five mortality reduction during the MDG period was the highest—32 per cent vis-à-vis 30 per cent among the remaining top five contributors put together (Figure 3.1). While the country should be lauded for this achievement, 11 per cent of total deaths in India still happen at the under-five level, comprising 19 per cent of all global under-five deaths—the figures for China being 2 and 3 per cent respectively (Figure 3.2). Indian policymakers can no longer hide behind the fact that India has a huge population and, therefore, smaller countries like Bangladesh, Nepal, Sri Lanka, and Maldives in its own vicinity—all of which performed much better than it—cannot be good examples. China, with a much bigger population until now, and lower GDP per capita (current USD) until 1990, has performed much better. In 1969, when dramatic declines in the number of under-five deaths in China began, its GDP per capita was 100 vis-à-vis 106 in India. Despite that, India had a much higher level of under-five mortality. A decade later, when China had recorded the world's highest level of decline in the number of under-five deaths, its GDP per capita was 184 and India did even better at 222 (World Development Indicators [WDI]). Bangladesh also demonstrated that growth in GDP per capita is not an indispensable condition for reductions in child mortality—it managed

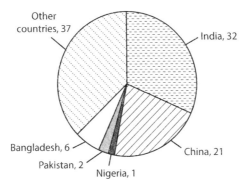

FIGURE 3.1   Decline in Under-Five Deaths among the Top Five Contributors to Under-Five Deaths (1990) and Other Countries as a Percentage of Global Decline in Under-Five Deaths, 1990 to 2015
Source: IGME.

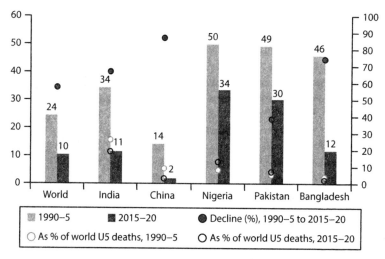

FIGURE 3.2   Under-Five Deaths as a Percentage of Total Deaths, World and
Top Five Contributors to Under-Five Deaths (1990), 1990–5 to 2015–20
Source: World Population Prospects: The 2017 Revision (WPP 2017), United
Nations, New York.
Note: U5 - Under-five. Bars map to the left axis, circles to the right.

a decline comparable to China's during the MDG era despite a much
lower increase in its GDP per capita vis-à-vis the latter's (Figure 3.3).

We often hear calls for increasing fiscal allocations to the health
sector in India, with policymakers and prominent economic advisers
arguing that we need economic growth and a wider tax base for the
government to have sufficient resources to be invested in health,
and existing allocations to the health sector need to be utilized with
greater efficiency and integrity. From the experience of China, India,
and Bangladesh, it seems that a commitment to child survival is more
important than either growth more broadly or allocations to the health
sector more particularly. In China, historic decline in mortality occurred
before free market reforms and lower GDP per capita vis-à-vis India. In
Bangladesh, not only has growth not been even closely as spectacular
as in India or China, its public expenditure on health (as a percentage of
GDP) actually got reduced from 1.2 to 0.8 per cent between 1995 and
2014—when substantial declines were happening in child mortality—
even as it increased from 1.1 to 1.4 per cent in India and 1.8 to 3.1 per cent
in China during this period (WDI). Sri Lanka is another case in India's

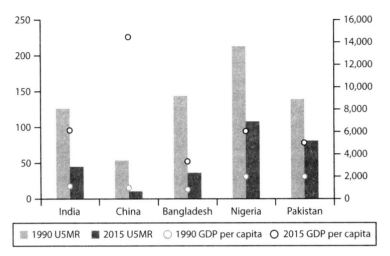

FIGURE 3.3   Changes in U5MR and GDP Per Capita (PPP, Current
International $) during MDG Era in Top Five Contributors, 1990 and 2015
Source: World Development Indicators (WDI), The World Bank.
Note: Bars map to the left axis, circles to the right.

neighbourhood where better health outcomes have been achieved with
concomitantly fewer allocations to the health sector. Clearly, a resourcist
approach to child mortality, as we discuss in greater detail in the next
chapters, is not very convincing as a central explanatory factor, while a
strong commitment to health and survival—which also perhaps leads to
greater efficiency and integrity in public health spending—seems more
plausible. The old English proverb, 'where there is a will, there is a way',
is also true for the allocation of higher resources for health. Health has
not been a political priority in India, nor have citizens considered health
or healthcare as a government obligation. Premature deaths, particularly
child deaths, therefore, have not been seen as a responsibility of the
government nor provoked any sense of injustice even among the otherwise vocal members of the civil society. What does the State owe its citizens, particularly to children, are questions which cannot be addressed in
such a context without invoking theories of justice—though not exclusively the ones discussed in political philosophy; certain religions, too,
for instance, have put forth principles, if not formal theories, of justice.

How have these countries done as far as the MDG 4 target (the reduction
in U5MR by two-thirds between 1990 and 2015) is concerned? Table 3.2

TABLE 3.2 Levels of Child Mortality (Rate) among Top Five Contributors to Global Under-Five Deaths (1990)

Country	1953	1969	1980	1990	2000	2010	2015	MDG 4 Target (2015)	Decline (%), 1990–2015
Under-Five Mortality Rate (U5MR)									
India	280	217	168	126	91	60	48	42	62
China		119	62	54	37	16	11	18	80
Nigeria		293	214	213	187	130	109	71	49
Pakistan	355	193	162	139	112	92	81	46	41
Bangladesh	323	225	199	144	88	50	38	48	74
Infant Mortality Rate (IMR)									
India	187	145	114	88	66	46	38	29	57
China		84	48	42	30	14	9	14	78
Nigeria		174	127	126	112	82	69	42	45
Pakistan	260	144	122	106	88	74	66	35	38
Bangladesh	217	150	134	100	64	39	31	33	69
Neonatal Mortality Rate (NNMR)									
India		85	72	57	45	33	28	19	52
China			54	30	21	8	6	10	81
Nigeria		69	71	50	48	38	34	17	32
Pakistan		75		64	60	50	46	21	29
Bangladesh		95	87	63	43	29	23	21	63

Source: IGME.

shows that Bangladesh and China surpassed their respective targets, with the former doing better despite being worse off than India in 1990 and earlier. India did not achieve its target, but did much better than Pakistan and Nigeria. Although not in our selection, India's neighbour Maldives was the best performer, not just in the region, but in the entire world—it recorded a reduction of 91 per cent between 1990 and 2015, with its U5MR declining from 94 to 9 during the MDG period. If we go back a bit further, its performance seems even more spectacular—in 1963, its U5MR of 324 was the ninth worst in the world, and worse than all countries in South Asia, with the sole exception of Afghanistan. Nepal and Bhutan, too, registering massive declines, achieved their MDG 4 targets in advance. Sri Lanka, widely known for its good record on health, could not meet the MDG 4 target and registered a decline of only 54 per cent, lower than India's. However, it started off from a threshold of 21 per cent that was even lower than China, and declines at those levels are more difficult since health systems have probably already reached their saturation levels in terms of existing capability. Even developed countries like Canada (with a decline of 41 per cent), US (42 per cent), Switzerland and France (52 per cent each) missed their targets, with New Zealand (49 per cent) performing slightly worse than Afghanistan (50 per cent). In all of these cases, we find that substantial declines from low thresholds are difficult. From a policy perspective, it highlights the problem of a *uniform* target for all countries, although a uniform target does reduce inter-country disparities (see Figure 5.1 in Chapter 5, for instance). This is discussed in more detail in Chapter 5.

Infant Deaths

Although our concern with child survival—and the well-being and future of children generally—should extend well beyond the age of five years, it would be helpful from a policy perspective to look at survival chances at lower levels, given variations in required interventions by these levels. For instance, it is considered that survival beyond the age of one year is more sensitive to socioeconomic rather than initial biomedical determinants—there is a detailed discussion of determinants in the next chapter. One might assume that justice might be a more relevant notion at the socioeconomic level—the term 'social' justice does convey that impression—but injustice could quite be at work at the biomedical level as well. We pick up this discussion in subsequent chapters in some detail. For now, let us get a quick sense of how India did vis-à-vis the top five contributors to under-five deaths at lower levels of child survival.

Declines in infant deaths were the primary drivers of declines in under-five mortality[3] in the MDG period in all countries except Nigeria, where child deaths were overwhelmingly responsible for gains made in reduction of under-five deaths (Figure 3.4). Paradoxically though, despite such gains in infant survival, infant deaths as a percentage of under-five deaths increased gradually in every country in our selection, especially in Bangladesh and India (Table 3.1). On the other hand, despite the lowest decline in infant deaths during the MDG period in Nigeria, infant deaths as a per cent of under-five deaths in 2015 were the lowest

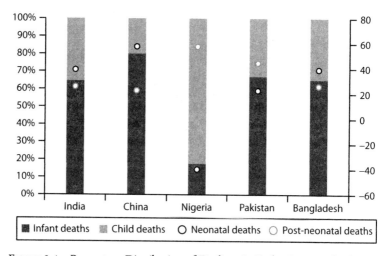

FIGURE 3.4   Percentage Distribution of Declines in Under-Five Deaths during the MDG Era in Top Five Contributors, 1990 and 2015
Source: IGME.
Note: Bars map to the left axis, circles to the right. Totals add up to 100 for infant (under 1 year) and child (1 to 5 year) deaths, collectively referred to as U5 deaths, and for neonatal (1st month since birth) and post-neonatal (1st to 12th month) deaths, collectively referred to as infant deaths.

[3] Under-five deaths can be broadly divided into infant and child deaths, and infant deaths into neonatal and post-neonatal deaths. See n 1 for the definitions of the various levels of child deaths.

among all—and despite the highest declines in China, the highest there. This implies that while other countries would have to continue their focus on infant mortality, Nigeria will have to focus on infant as well as child mortality. As far as the MDG 4 target of infant mortality rate is concerned, the situation is similar to that in U5MR—while China and Bangladesh surpassed their targets, India, Nigeria, and Pakistan missed them, the latter two quite seriously (Table 3.2).

Neonatal Deaths

Declines in infant deaths were further largely driven by declines in neo-natal deaths, again with the exception of Nigeria and Pakistan, where declines in post-neonatal deaths were more prominent. While Nigeria actually registered a 20 per cent increase in the number of neonatal deaths during the MDG period, China recorded a massive decline of 90 per cent and was the only country with a decline in neonatal deaths as a per cent of infant deaths. Despite a 55 per cent decline in the number of neonatal deaths, India still accounted for 26 per cent of all neonatal deaths in the world in the year 2015. Its BIMARU (sick) states—Bihar, Madhya Pradesh (MP), Rajasthan and Uttar Pradesh (UP)—accounted for 55 per cent of neonatal deaths in the country—10, 10, 8, and 27 per cent respectively—or 15 per cent of the total global burden in 2011 (Zodpey and Paul 2014).

As far as the neonatal mortality rate (NNMR) is concerned, China did exceptionally better than other countries as well as its own perfor-mance at higher levels of child deaths, and was the only country that achieved the MDG 4 target in NNMR. On the contrary, not only did India miss its target, its performance was worse than at the under-five and infant levels. Bangladesh could not make it to its target in this case, but did, however, register the second highest decline.

Early neonatal mortality is death within the first week of birth. International data and attention on this level of child mortality has been scarce, let alone on day one mortality, which constitutes a substantial portion of early neonatal deaths. According to the WHO and UNICEF estimates, 2.8 million deaths in 2004, or 76 per cent of total neonatal deaths, happened at the early neonatal level. In India, nearly 45 per cent of under-five deaths or 73 per cent of neonatal deaths happened at this level. Thirty-seven per cent of neonatal deaths or nearly 60 per cent of early neonatal deaths occurred on day one, as per NFHS-3 (Padmadas et al. 2013; UNICEF 2008a, 2008b; Zodpey and Paul 2014).[4]

One set of literature[5] argued that because an increasing proportion of under-five deaths were concentrated at the neonatal level, MDG 4's U5MR target 'cannot be met without substantial reductions in neonatal mortality'. This may not hold in all cases. To begin with, let us look at China, where it did seem to hold—declines in neonatal mortality were the highest compared to other levels (Table 3.1), even as the contribution of decline in neonatal deaths to under-five deaths was also the highest (Figure 3.4). However, both India and Bangladesh registered a decline of 39 per cent in neonatal mortality during the MDG era (Figure 3.4), yet the latter achieved its MDG target in U5MR while the former could not. Not only that, neonatal deaths in Bangladesh as a percentage of infant deaths are slightly higher than in India, which means it would have to focus more on the neonatal level despite having achieved the MDG 4 target in U5MR. Nigeria's case is more divergent—to achieve its MDG 4 target in U5MR, Nigeria would have to focus almost equally on all levels of under-five deaths, and not disproportionately on the neonatal.

At the global level, while neonatal deaths as a percentage of under-five deaths went up from 40 to 45 per cent during the MDG period[6]—and could further go up to 52 per cent by the end of the

---

[4] For a discussion on the trends, determinants and inequalities in early neonatal mortality in India using Sample Registration System (SRS) and National Family Health Survey (NFHS) data, see Jena (2012).

[5] Arokiasamy and Gautam (2008); Hill and Choi (2006); ICMR (2007); Lawn, Cousens, and Zupan (2005); Lawn et al. (2009); Oestergaard et al. (2011); Pandey et al. (2005); WHO (2006).

[6] Given that 98 per cent of neonatal deaths are concentrated in the developing world, the global increase in neonatal deaths as a percentage of under-five deaths mirrors the increase in such deaths in the developing regions from 40 to 45 per cent during the MDG period. The corresponding increase in developed regions was 52 per cent to 55 per cent (IGME 2015), which means that this is more of a global phenomenon, although its causes in developed and developing countries could be very different. In the latter, it might mean saturation of the limits of preventability since they offer better access not just to healthcare but also the broader determinants of health. Likewise, in developing countries too, early deaths cannot just be addressed through healthcare alone. We discuss this in detail later.

SDG era in 2030—almost half of deaths will still occur at the higher under-five levels. Although from a moral perspective, the earlier the death the more intolerable it is, we should not further *reduce* the focus of survival from the under-five to the neonatal—or further to the first day and week, where most of the neonatal deaths are concentrated—from a policy perspective. This is not an argument against priority to early deaths, but against a reductionist and funnel-ling-down approach to survival in general, child survival in particu-lar. Further, given the interconnections of even early survival with maternal nutritional and health status—and thereby with the larger determinants of health, as we discuss later—a reduction in focus to neonatal deaths does not imply priority to biomedical vis-à-vis struc-tural determinants or interventions of survival, if that is what the advocates of this literature are trying to drive ahead. The rhetoric in India has already changed dramatically toward medical interventions like vaccinations—not surprisingly though, given that it is world's leading hub of vaccine manufacturing—missing out completely on the broader socioeconomic dynamics that continue to keep child mortality a lively challenge.

To take this argument further, while primary healthcare systems have a central role to play in the health and survival of the child and the mother, it would be unjust to place the bulk of responsibility on them. One of the reasons why primary health systems in developing countries like India are overburdened and inefficient is because they are expected to address problems arising out of economic or educa-tion systems, for instance. Individuals from economically and educa-tionally weaker households have higher chances of falling sick, being malnourished and dying early, and healthcare systems are expected to compensate for shortfalls in these structural conditions. Justice is about justified expectations and allocation of responsibilities among various actors. An important question regarding the appropriate focus on the level of mortality is—what do governments owe to their citi-zens: primary or prolonged as well as decent survival? This relates to the question we raised at the very beginning of this book—what do we owe our children? We need to broaden rather than reduce our concern with human survival, both quantitatively (in terms of life expectancy) and qualitatively (in terms of quality of life). Only when we see child survival as a problem of justice can this happen. Child survival is not just about primary healthcare for the child and mother, it is about justice for them in particular—more particularly the child—and in the wider society at large.

Intra-Country Comparisons

While the aggregate child mortality indicators in India are, as briefly discussed earlier, not quite encouraging, as in several other aspects, there are considerable variations within the country at different levels of disaggregation. To begin with, under-five deaths as a per cent of total deaths in 2015 ranged from 3 per cent in Kerala to 22 in Bihar (Figure 3.5). Internationally, only 0.3 per cent of deaths in Japan happened at this level, while in Canada, United States, and Sri Lanka, these figures were 0.8, 1.1, and 2.5 per cent respectively (UNPD 2015). As expected, BIMARU states accounted for 57 per cent of all under-five deaths in India in 2012—UP leading the group with 28 per cent of the total (Figure 3.6). Given that these states have been backward on account of various socioeconomic

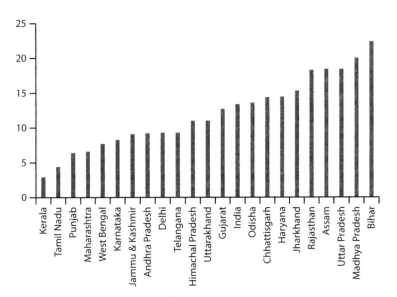

FIGURE 3.5   Under-Five Deaths as a Percentage of Total Deaths, India and Major States, 2015
Source: SRS.

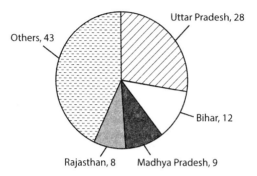

FIGURE 3.6   Under-Five Deaths as a Percentage of Total National Deaths in BIMARU and Other States, 2012
Source: Ram et al. 2013.

indicators demonstrates that child mortality is not just a biomedical but a broader socioeconomic challenge, with injustice playing a major role beyond aggregate inefficiencies and injustices. All BIMARU states, particularly UP, are dens of social injustice, and it clearly shows in their aggregate as well as disaggregated performance, as discussed later.

Figure 3.7 depicts how selected Indian states and union territories (UTs) have performed as per four rounds of DHS or NFHS,[7] as the DHS are christened in India. With the highest number of under-five deaths and the highest U5MR as well during the NFHS-1 and NFHS-4 reference periods, it is clear that UP was largely responsible for keeping India back from achieving its MDG 4 target. In August 2017, the deaths of more than a hundred children in a government hospital in its Gorakhpur district—represented by the state's chief minister, Yogi Adityanath, in the national Parliament since 1998–9—brought the issue of child deaths under media limelight. However, within a few days, the issue was no more a public concern, with the state government persistently arguing that the parents of the dead children rather than the state were responsible. While UP did better in terms of decline vis-à-vis

[7] NFHS-1: 1992–3; NFHS-2: 1998–9; NFHS-3: 2005–6; NFHS-4: 2014–15. 'The figures of NFHS-4 and that of earlier rounds may not be strictly comparable due to differences in sample size and NFHS-4 will be a benchmark for future surveys', says the India factsheet of the NFHS-4 in its introduction.

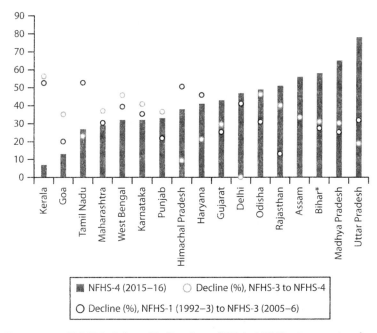

FIGURE 3.7   U5MR in Selected Indian States/UTs in NFHS-4 (2015–16) and
Declines (%) between NFHS-1 to NFHS-3 and NFHS-3 to NFHS-4
Source: NFHS state/UT reports (NFHS-1 to NFHS-3), NFHS factsheets (NFHS-4).
Note: Declines between NFHS-1 and -3 were calculated using data from respective
NFHS state/UT reports and was for the ten-year period preceding the survey.
Declines between NFHS-3 and NFHS-4 were calculated using data from NFHS-4
factsheets (full data or reports were not available at the time of writing) and was
for the five-year period preceding the survey. *Bihar includes Jharkhand from
NFHS-1 to NFHS-3, but not in declines between NFHS-3 and NFHS-4.

economically prosperous states like Punjab, Gujarat, and Maharashtra
between NFHS-1 and NFHS-3, its performance was average, with health-
advanced states like Kerala and Tamil Nadu being the top performers,
recording declines of 53 per cent each. Between NFHS-3 and NFHS-4
too, Kerala was the top-performer, with an improved decline of 56 per
cent. However, Tamil Nadu slipped to the bottom of the list with a mea-
gre decline of 23 per cent, slightly better than UP's 19 per cent, which,
in turn, did only better than Himachal Pradesh and Delhi. It is surprising that Delhi recorded a nil decline during the last decade—in NFHS-3,

it was just behind Tamil Nadu; by NFHS-4, it was not only way behind
the latter, but worse than a state like Haryana and only slightly better
than Odisha, one of the poorest states in the country. If Kerala stands
out for its continued progress and lead over other states for decades,
Rajasthan—and, to an extent, Odisha, Goa, and Punjab—are examples
of how child survival can be improved within a decade. On the other
hand, states like Himachal Pradesh, Delhi, Tamil Nadu, and Haryana
are examples of how the momentum of progress can slow down over
time, and likewise the importance of keeping issues like child survival
on priority on a regular basis. As we argue later, states should not stop
until they reach zero preventable mortality—that level also needs to be
maintained with persistent efforts over time, a lesson for even states like
Kerala. It is not just about reaching an international or national target
on child survival—it is about zero tolerance for any preventable child
death and, beyond that, enhancing the conditions of survival. Before
we move on, let us quickly add that while northeastern states such as
Nagaland, Mizoram, Meghalaya, and Arunachal Pradesh were not in
our selection, their situation had actually worsened between NFHS-1
and NFHS-3, and yet none of them were part of the Empowered Action
Group (EAG) states,[8] which means performance over time was not a
consideration as far as the policy focus was concerned. In particular,
Arunachal Pradesh had a much worse U5MR in NFHS-3 than even
Uttaranchal, still the latter was part of EAG states, but not the former.
The selection seems to have been largely based on aggregative rather
than equity considerations.[9] Arunachal Pradesh went on to record the

[8] EAG was constituted in 2001 by the Government of India (GoI)—
comprising the GoI's Ministry of Health and Family Welfare (MoHFW) and
other relevant ministries as well as state governments—to prepare, implement
and monitor area specific health interventions in 284 districts from Assam and
8 states with the highest levels of child mortality—BIMARU states, Chhattisgarh,
Jharkhand, Odisha, and Uttarakhand. To facilitate district-level planning and
progress monitoring, the Annual Health Surveys (AHS) were launched by the
GoI, which went on for three years, but were later discontinued since NFHS-4
was going to provide data at the district level.

[9] 'These nine states, which account for about 48 per cent of the total population in the country, are the high-focus states in view of their relatively higher
fertility and mortality indicators' (AHS press release, 10 August 2011).

highest decline (63 per cent), better than even Kerala, between NFHS-3 and NFHS-4—that too, with lowest immunization coverage among Indian states/UTs in NFHS-3 (24 per cent of its children aged between 12 and 23 months received no vaccination), and the second worst after Mizoram in NFHS-4 (20 per cent). So much for the omnipotent power of vaccines! Not just U5MR, this did not prevent it from having one of the lowest infant mortality rates (IMRs) in NFHS-4 either. Making healthcare the central axis of equality is a risky proposition, to say the least, as we elaborate in the next chapters.

As far as the performance of major Indian states vis-à-vis their specific MDG 4 IMR targets[10] are concerned, we see in Figure 3.8 that Tamil Nadu is the only state that achieved and slightly outperformed

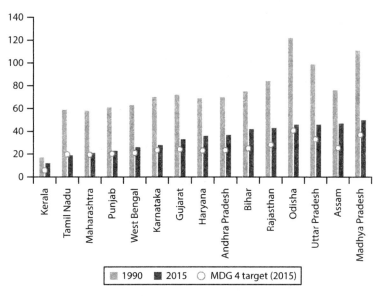

FIGURE **3.8**   IMR in Selected States and IMR MDG 4 Target, 2015
Source: SRS.

[10]   IMR is the second indicator under MDG 4. Since we only have IMR estimates for India and states for the MDG reference year, 1990, we have used IMR here. While discussion of MDGs have been confined to national levels, it has been argued that such targets can also be calculated, and should be used to assess performance, at subnational levels (World Bank 2004: 6).

its target. Even Kerala missed its target. Kerala, in fact, had the lowest percentage decline (29 per cent) in IMR between 1990 and 2015, while Tamil Nadu had the highest (68 per cent). Although BIMARU and other laggard states like Assam and Haryana did not expectedly do well, Odisha's performance was unexpectedly the third best (62 per cent), which is remarkable given its low socioeconomic performance vis-à-vis most Indian states/UTs, although its IMR was also the third worst in 2015 (46). Kerala's IMR is still the lowest in the country, and Tamil Nadu is still not even where Kerala was in 1990, so both Tamil Nadu as well as Kerala need to continue with their focus on child survival. Kerala's case supports the argument that declines at lower levels of child mortality have been slower, and the importance of a continued focus on child survival—and moving to higher-order measures of child well-being and flourishing. Nevertheless, while only a third of infant deaths were concentrated at the early neonatal level in Kerala, it was more than 50 per cent among the major states and as high as 63 per cent in the fragile state of Jammu and Kashmir (J&K) (SRS 2013).[11] We revisit the latter in the further sections in the context of life expectancy at birth and higher ages.

Regarding neonatal mortality rate (Figure 3.9), Tamil Nadu was, once again, the only state that reached its MDG 4 target by recording the highest decline (68 per cent) between 1990 and 2015. Kerala, once again, missed the mark with a decline of 52 per cent, equal to that of UP, and slightly worse than that of MP and Odisha. Nevertheless, once again, Kerala had the lowest NNMR in 2015, while Tamil Nadu continues to be more than 25 years behind. Both of them need to keep their momentum, more so Kerala. Where Kerala's performance was the highest (U5MR), we still have high inter-state differentials; where its performance was moderate (NNMR) to lowest (IMR), such differentials

[11] The SRS is the world's largest demographic survey, covering a population of 7.3 million across Indian states and UTs, conducted under the aegis of the Office of the Registrar General of India (RGI), Ministry of Home Affairs (MHA), Government of India, providing reliable estimates of fertility and mortality at the national and state level on a regular basis since 1971. For a detailed overview of mortality statistics sources and their reporting status in India, refer to GoI (2007) and GoI (2009). We use mortality statistics from various rounds of SRS, NFHS as well as the National Sample Surveys (NSS).

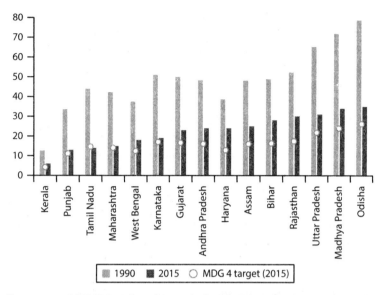

FIGURE 3.9   NNMR in Selected States and NNMR MDG 4 Target, 2015
Source: SRS.

have gone down substantially. Not that Kerala is responsible for them—
many of the backward states did quite well on these indicators—but the
policy and philosophical question is: should such reduction in inequalities at the inter-state level be celebrated? Should policy focus be decided
based on low current status or also on low performance over time? Such
questions also emerge when we discuss inter-group inequalities in child
survival later in this chapter. We discuss their policy and philosophical
implications in the final chapter. For now, it is important to note that,
contrary to the argument that declines at the neonatal level have been
lower—which is why India could not achieve its MDG 4 national target
on U5MR—does not seem to be true. Declines during the MDG period
ranged from 38 to 68 per cent in NNMR, 29 to 68 per cent for IMR, and
13 to 51 per cent between NFHS-1 and NFHS-3 and 0 to 56 per cent
between NFHS-3 and NFHS-4 in the case of U5MR.

Before moving on to inter-group differentials in child survival, let
us discuss an interesting case of life expectancy in Kerala and J&K,
according to figures put out by SRS 2015. Figure 3.10 shows that with
its moderate record on child mortality, J&K was behind Kerala in life

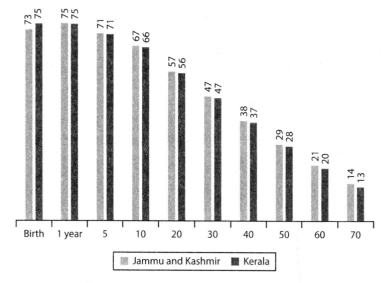

FIGURE 3.10   Life Expectancy at Various Age Levels in Jammu and Kashmir and Kerala, 2010–14
Source: SRS.

expectancy at birth (LEB). Nevertheless, it gains an advantage over Kerala and becomes the state with the highest life expectancy in the country at most higher age groups, despite being the country's most fragile state, particularly since 1989 when prolonged militancy began there. In the next chapter, we discuss how these states are placed on access to various determinants of health. In the final chapters, we discuss their policy and philosophical implications. It is quite ironic that a state in which survival is most precarious, life expectancy is the highest.

Group Differentials

Let us now discuss differentials in child survival among social groups within as well as across states. Not just from an equity perspective, inter-group inequalities could be important from an efficiency perspective too where inequalities are pervasive and entrenched, as they are in India. One could argue that pervasive and entrenched injustice has been the biggest structural factor responsible for persistently high levels of child mortality in the country—it has not only ensured deprivations in some of the worst forms, it has not allowed a unified public voice to emerge in favour of such a fundamental human right like child survival to emerge. However, before we go ahead, let us provide a quick justification for focusing on inter-group differentials as we argued earlier in favour of an individual focus and there is a body of literature—though more prominent in income rather than in health inequality measurement—that argues for focusing on individuals rather than groups in inequality measurement at a broader level.

Individual or Group Inequality

Let us start out by saying that, unless further disaggregated, group inequalities frame individuals within concerned groups in a simplistic framework—rich or poor, for instance. A rich or a poor individual could be many other things at the same time, and by only taking his income or wealth status, we are ignoring other aspects of their case. A rich person may have a higher proneness to ill health than a poor individual, and we would have to ask whether a health policy should ignore him just because he is rich. This is particularly relevant in the case of child deaths among otherwise socioeconomically privileged households. What should be the primary criterion for prioritization in health—health, wealth, or some other background characteristic? Prioritization is not always about the allocation of limited healthcare resources, and making resource-allocation or affordability a central concern of health policy emanates from a resourcist approach to health and health justice. Wider socioeconomic inequities have a bearing on health status and healthcare affordability, but one could argue that in matters of health policy, health outcomes should be of primary concern, and the economics of healthcare or other variables secondary. Applying a *social* or group justice approach to health policy leads to confusion in health priorities. At the most primary level, health inequalities should be about inequalities in health outcomes, full stop, irrespective of the background of individuals. In the measurement of individual inequality in health outcomes, the focus is squarely on health per se, which is intuitively quite appealing. And, as we noted at the beginning of the book, the politics and practice of social justice seems to benefit select individuals from target groups, while the rest from within that group as well as deserving individuals from outside the group are neglected. This is the concern that led to the central question of this book—what should be the central variable on the basis of which justice and equality should be pursued and measured?

From our perspective, a concern with inequality should start—not end—with the broadest level (inequality between nations, which is what international development goals like the MDGs and SDGs have been essentially concerned about, for instance) and go down to the individual level. There are structural determinants of health which affect aggregates at a broader level—outdoor air pollution in north India being the most vivid example—and it would make sense to measure their health impact and address them at an aggregate rather than at an individual level. Although Sunita Narain, a highly prominent Indian environmentalist, looks at air pollution as 'a great equalizer',[12] it would still make sense to look at inequality in the health impact of outdoor air pollution at an individual level—some individuals have the awareness and affordability to buy air purifiers for their houses and use masks when outside, while others do not. Nevertheless, the notion and practice of 'public' health is based on a broad structural understanding of health, and the absence of effective aggregate interventions will only lead to or worsen individual inequalities in health. This corresponds with Sen's notion of 'effective freedoms', as discussed in the previous chapter. Aggregates do not always have to be geographical—such as countries, states, districts, and localities—they can also be defined socioeconomically, by gender, caste, religion, and so on. Also, with increasing prevalence of non-communicable diseases (NCDs), there is a stronger case for public health to go beyond its traditional geographical focus and look at other such aggregates, as far as their socioeconomic, cultural and other larger risk factors are concerned.

Discrimination is another reality that has a distinctly group-based dimension and can reflect in health outcomes both directly and indirectly—from the provision and access to healthcare to broader socioeconomic and political spheres. Many a time, we do not like particular individuals—irrespective of their background—and discriminate against them, but such discrimination is difficult to show up in individual health inequalities,

---

[12] *Hindustan Times*, 'Excerpt: Conflicts of Interest by Sunita Narain', 24 November 2017.

contrary to group-based health inequities which have systematic and persistent patterns. So, as we observe in this and the next chapter, both aggregate public as well as group-based discriminations are relevant for considerations of justice—the former relates to structural injustice, with implications for entire populations, irrespective of background, though in variable degrees, and the latter to social injustice against specific group of individuals.

Nevertheless, although we can start with aggregate inequalities, the effort should be to go down as deep as possible. For instance, we can start out with Dalits as a broad category, but then go ahead and study how poor Dalits or Dalit women are doing. Within Dalit women, how are the educated and uneducated or poor and rich doing? Injustice is complex and we need to treat it in that manner. The central focal variable of justice has to be sensitive to such complexity. This complexity in the measurement of inequality does not end with the level at which it should be measured. Even when we agree to look at group-based inequalities, we need to decide whom to compare with whom (the issue of the 'comparator' or reference group, which we would pick up in the final chapter), the time horizon (should we only look at inequality in the present or in performance over time as well) and, perhaps most importantly, in terms of actual achievements or vis-à-vis the distance from the potentials of respective groups and individuals. We will take up these more complex issues in the final chapter, and move on to a discussion of group-based inequalities in various combinations, some of them unusual, at the moment.

A Note on Data

While we have tried to present relevant data by background characteristics from a host of reliable—including some rare historical—sources, for several domains, to ensure that observed trends are longitudinally as well as latitudinally sound, it is primarily meant to be illustrative rather than exhaustive, to serve the purpose of aiding the broader policy and normative discussions that the book is concerned with. Further research utilizing newer or more refined data is welcome to take the discussion forward. Second, I have restricted myself to the data given in printed reports, which anyone can freely access and use for cross-verification, rather than go by calculations from raw data, which I feel, leaves non-statisticians with no option but to accept it at face value. This again is not a problem as far as the purpose of our empirical consideration is concerned.

Reliable gender-based data on IMR has been available since 1958 (NSS 14th round), and has been provided by SRS since 1961. SRS also conducted three special mortality surveys, and provided data by caste, religion, and so on for the first time in 1978,[13] and later in 1984 and 1997.[14] On a more comparable basis, we have various levels of child mortality rates from three rounds of NFHS.[15] Indirect child mortality estimates by these background characteristics are also available from Census of India 1981, 1991, 2001 (not yet from Census 2011), but since these years are already covered either by SRS or NFHS surveys, we have not included them here. We have also not included child mortality data from non-governmental sources, for example, India Human Development Survey (IHDS),[16] since available data was already covered by NFHS-3. Official child mortality statistics are based on larger sample sizes, hence more representative than most non-governmental surveys at the national level at least. Data has been presented by three major axes of social injustice—gender, tribe/caste, religion—for India and one state from each region (North, South, East, West, Central India) with the highest percentage of STs as per NFHS-3—since their population is, in most cases, the lowest—to capture regional variations as well.

---

[13] Seventy-seven per cent of India's population was rural as per Census 1981, so rural IMR is a fair representation of overall IMR, which was not uniformly available across these special surveys. U5MR figures were also not available in these as in most other SRS surveys.

[14] It is only for recent years that we have SRS data on U5MR. In 1978 SRS special survey, we had rural and urban, but not total, IMR; in 1984 and 1997 special surveys, total IMR was also given. For comparability purposes, we only took rural IMR for all these three years. This was not a problem by gender, so we took total IMR in that case. NFHS had both IMR and U5MR for all groups, so we took the latter, which is more sensitive to socioeconomic determinants, and hence more relevant for our particular case.

[15] We could have included NFHS-4 data for inter-group differentials as we did for the states, and compared NFHS-1 to NFHS-3 and NFHS-3 to NFHS-4 differentials separately. However, since this work does not aspire to be an update of latest data, we decided against doing that.

[16] IHDS (IHDS-1: 2004–5; IHDS-2: 2011–12, data not available yet), have been jointly conducted by the University of Maryland (US) and the New Delhi-based National Council of Applied Economic Research (NCAER).

Historical Data

Gender

Inequality can be measured using a variety of comparators—if only to bring out its complexity and make the discussion more interesting using non-traditional approaches. We will do it here. However, let us begin with a historical view of how the traditional binary differentials in child survival have evolved in the country and gain insights on inequality as a dynamic process.

Females are said to have a biological advantage in survival, reflected in child survival and life expectancy data in most parts of the world. That used to be the case in most parts of India too. However, over time, females lost their biological advantage in survival. During 1958–9 (Figure 3.11),[17] rural IMR was lower among females with a few

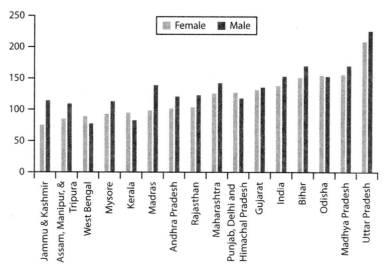

FIGURE **3.11**   Rural IMR by Gender, India and Selected States, 1958–9
Source: NSS 14th Round, Report No. 76 (Fertility and Mortality Rates in India), Cabinet Secretariat: GoI, 1963.

[17] NSS 7th round (1953–4) also provided rural IMR at the all-India level (173 for males, 129 for females), but the sample size was quite small, hence it has not been included here. During the NSS 14th round (1958–9) too, which we have included here, only rural IMR was available for India and erstwhile states. From

exceptions, in cases dramatically lower (for example, in the erstwhile provinces of Madras and J&K). What is surprising is that it was lower even in the BIMARU states—despite Bihar, MP, and UP being at the bottom as usual—but actually higher in Kerala, where both male and female IMRs were worse than West Bengal. Figure 3.12 shows that female IMR was nowhere worse than male IMR in 1961—equal in Rajasthan, which is actually the worst case in the selection, and way much lower than male IMR in West Bengal.[18] However, lower improvement over

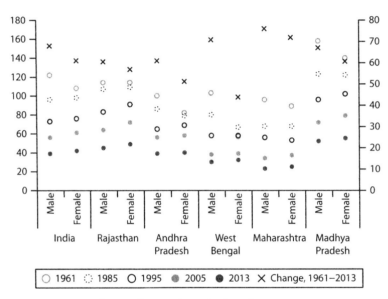

FIGURE 3.12   IMR by Gender in India and Selected States, 1961–2013
Source: SRS.
Note: Circles map to the left axis, crosses to the right. In the case of West Bengal females, the circles of 1961 and 1995 almost overlap—the respective values were 57 and 58 respectively.

_____

the 19th round (1964–5), we have national level IMRs for rural and urban areas—it was 119 and 110 in rural India, 89 and 70 in urban India for males and females respectively. For a brief history of infant mortality statistics in India from the early period until the 1970s, see Chandrasekhar (1972: 73–6).

[18] The variation between 1958–9 and 1961 data for West Bengal could possibly be due to the fact that the former is for rural areas only, while the latter for rural and urban areas combined.

time meant that female IMR became higher than males in all cases by 2013. Evidence from DHS surveys is similar—even countries in sub-Saharan Africa had female survival advantage, which kept worsening in India over time (Figure 3.13). U5MR from the Census of India 1981, 1991, and 2001 reveals the same picture—female U5MR was 6.8 per cent higher than male U5MR in 1981, and this increased to 11 and 21.8 per cent in 1991 and 2001 respectively. The biological underpinnings of female advantage and the social underpinnings of disadvantage in South Asia are evident in Figure 3.14—females continue to have an advantage at the neonatal level, which starts disappearing as they survive more and more.

Likewise, females in India had higher life expectancy at birth at the beginning of the twentieth century, but they lost their advantage, to regain it in the 1980s (Figure 3.15). However, female advantage has been minuscule—no wonder aggregate life expectancy at birth in the country in 2015 (68 years) was not only lower vis-à-vis Maldives (77 years), Sri Lanka (75 years), Bangladesh (72 years), and Bhutan and Nepal (70 years each) in its neighbourhood, but also highly fragile countries

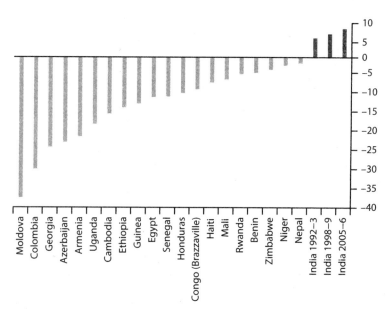

FIGURE 3.13   Percentage Higher/Lower Female U5MR vis-à-vis Male U5MR in India and Other DHS Countries, 2005/2006
Source: Demographic and Health Surveys (DHS).

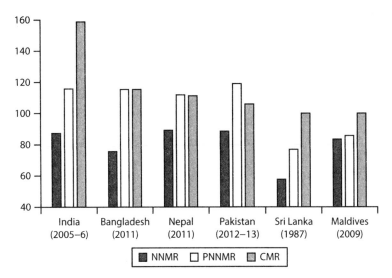

FIGURE **3.14**   Percent Higher/Lower Female vs Male NNMR, PNNMR, and CMR in India and DHS South Asian Countries

Source: DHS.

Note: 100, less than 100, and more than 100 means equal, lower, and higher female rate vis-a-vis the male rate, respectively.

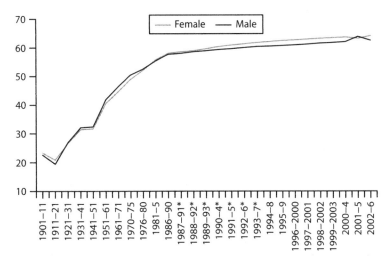

FIGURE **3.15**   Life Expectancy at Birth (in Years) by Gender, India, 1901–2006

* Excludes the state of Jammu and Kashmir.

Source: RGI.

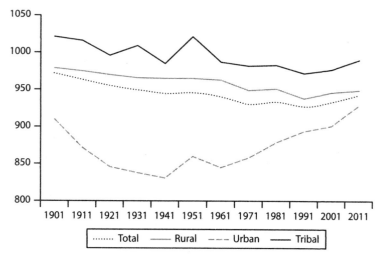

FIGURE **3.16**   Sex Ratio in India, Census 1901–2011
Source: Maharatna (2011) and Census of India (2011).

like the West Bank and Gaza (73 years), Iraq and Syria (70 years) (WDI).
Another related indicator is the sex ratio, which too tells us the same
story. Sex ratio in general (Figure 3.16), and child sex ratio in particular
(Figure 3.17), declined over the decades, with the former recording

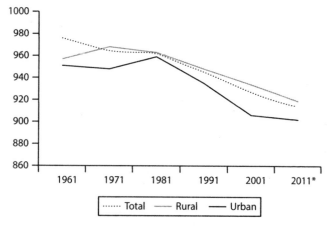

FIGURE **3.17**   Child Sex Ratio (0–6 Years) in India, Census 1961 to 2011
* Based on provisional population totals.
Source: Census (2011) (Provisional Population Totals) and RGI (2011).

some improvement since 1991. Nevertheless, while urban India's sex ratio has been improving since 1961, rural India experienced a steady decline until 1991, narrowing the rural-urban divide. Is such inequality reduction to be celebrated? Tribal sex ratio has not only been better than the national average, but also than the rural on a continuous basis. We will talk about tribal female advantage later—although there has been decline in this advantage over time, thanks to increasing mainstream influence on tribal society. Child sex ratio, on the other hand, has persistently declined over the past few census decades, especially since 1981. The Central as well as several state governments have been taking steps to tackle it, but not with much success overall—there were only four districts in the entire country in 2011 with a child sex ratio over 1000—Lahaul and Spiti (1013) in Himachal Pradesh; Tawang (1005) in Arunachal Pradesh; Dakshin Bastar Dantewada (1005) in Chhattisgarh; and Aizawl (1003) in Mizoram. On a positive note, two neighbouring states with the worst records on child sex ratio, Punjab and Haryana, registered improvement from 798 and 819 in Census 2001 to 846 and 830 in Census 2011 respectively. Yet, another neighbouring state, J&K, recorded the worst change during this period—from 941 to 859.

Figure 3.18 shows how child sex ratio worsens with improvement in economic and educational status in India. It has been argued that education and wealth bring about better awareness and access to sex-selection technology (prenatal discrimination) vis-à-vis rural, poorer, and uneducated sections of the population that traditionally resort to postnatal discrimination (female infanticide to a much lesser extent now, but bias against female children in access to healthcare, nutrition, and so on is still quite pervasive). Demographers have pointed out to the latter as the principal determinant of low sex ratio until the late 1980s (Arokiasamy 2007),[19] while this dubious distinction now belongs to the former, thanks to fertility declines due to improvements in educational and economic status, population stabilization measures, and so on in the context of persistent son preference. This is one of the aspects of contemporary India that demonstrates the continuing strength of traditional biases, and highlights the significance of focusing

[19] For an annotated review of literature on declining child sex ratio in India, see CDS and UNFPA 2009 (*Declining Child Sex Ratio (0–6 years) in India: A Review of Literature and Annotated Bibliography*).

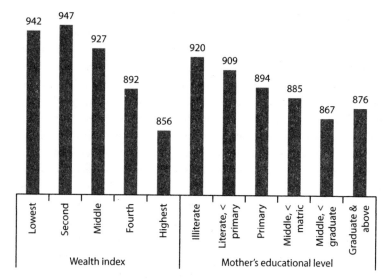

FIGURE **3.18** Child Sex Ratio by Wealth Index for 5-year Period Preceding the Survey (NFHS-3) and Sex Ratio at Birth by Mother's Education Level (Census 2001), India
Source: IIPS 2009.

on non-institutional dimensions for a just policy of child survival. There are institutional mechanisms in place to check them, but people have found ways to evade them, as happens more generally in the country. From an empirical perspective, higher wealth and education—considered determinants of better child survival—can also become reverse determinants when it comes to child sex ratio in India.

Coming back to under-five mortality, with a slightly different lens, Figure 3.19 discusses gender differentials in U5MR by residence. Although Kerala did better than all other states in the aggregate, it has the highest level of female disadvantage in U5MR at the urban level and worse than most states at total and rural levels, if we are to go by estimates provided by SRS. Given Kerala's low mortality rates, this only means a differential of 3 in the urban context (male U5MR was 7 and female 10). However, even if we were to go by differential in terms of numbers rather than proportion, even BIMARU states such as Bihar (with a differential of −2), MP (0), and UP (−2) do better than Kerala in urban areas. The potential of U5MR as an indicator of social

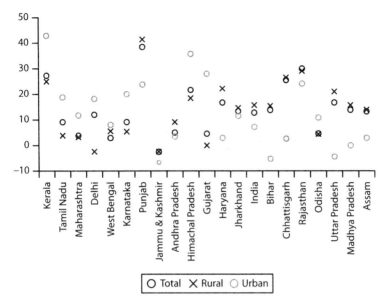

Figure 3.19   Female–Male Percentage Differentials in U5MR by Residence, India and Major States/UTs, 2013
Source: SRS.

development seems doubtful, at least as far as these numbers are concerned, given that we know otherwise what the gender situation is in these states. With the exception of J&K, females in all states have higher U5MR than males at the aggregate level. And we just indicated above that this was a state which recorded the worst change in child sex ratio between 2001 and 2011.

There is another way of looking at differentials—for instance, how urban males are doing vis-à-vis rural males, and how urban females are doing vis-à-vis rural females. Figure 3.20 shows that general differentials between urban and rural U5MR (there is higher percentage of U5MR in rural areas) ranges from 28 to 126 per cent in Himachal Pradesh and Assam respectively. With lower levels of socioeconomic development and access to healthcare in rural areas, such differentials are widely recognized, although at the aggregate national level, they have been continuously declining over the decades. However, the huge differentials among males and females by type of residence are not well known. Himachal Pradesh and Assam also have the lowest and highest

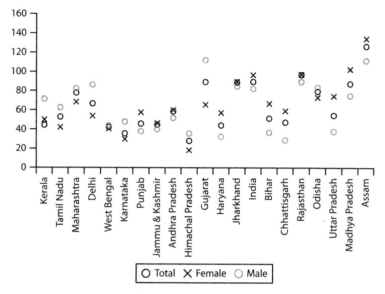

FIGURE 3.20   Rural–Urban Percentage Differentials in U5MR by Gender,
India and Major States/UTs, 2013
Source: SRS 2013.

differentials among females by residence, while in the case of males, it is Gujarat with the lowest and Chhattisgarh (one of the economically most and least developed states in the country) with the highest. Assam stands with Gujarat on male differentials by residence. What is also interesting is that in several states, it is actually the rural–urban male differential which is higher than rural–urban female differential. If we are to consider this from a policy perspective, we cannot stop at rural–urban differentials, but also disaggregate further by gender and other axes for which data is (or should be made) available. And, from the principles of justice as discussed in political philosophy, do we give preference to the male differentials by type of residence since they are higher than the female differentials?

As mentioned earlier, we should try to consider as disaggregated a data as available/possible. Figures 3.21 and 3.22 offer us a glimpse of U5MR by gender and residence among two major religious groups— Hindus and Muslims—from Census 1981 and among the scheduled castes (SCs), scheduled tribes (STs) as well as at the aggregate level from

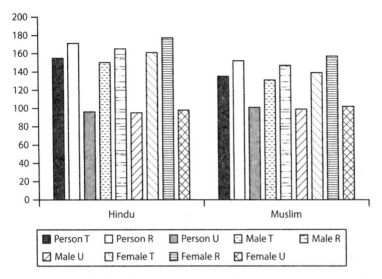

FIGURE 3.21   U5MR by Religion, Gender, and Residence, Census 1981, India
Source: RGI 1988.
Note: T = Total, R = Rural, U = Urban.

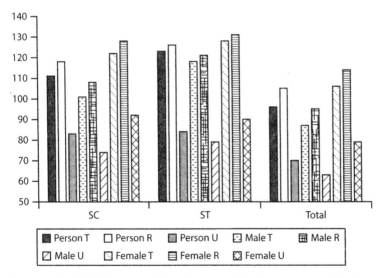

FIGURE 3.22   U5MR by Caste / Tribe, Gender, and Residence, Census 2001, India
Source: RGI 2009a.
Note: T = Total, R = Rural, U = Urban.

Census 2001 respectively. Urban males perform better across all groups, reflecting gender and urban bias cutting across caste/tribe as well as religion. Female disadvantage is a highly pervasive problem in the country, and therefore needs to be addressed on top priority, across all groups. However, contrary to the broader pattern, according to which Muslims have had an advantage in child survival, as we observe further, and which is also reflected here as well—on the whole, Muslims did way much better than Hindus—Hindu urban males and females performed better than their Muslim counterparts. The Hindu average vis-à-vis the Muslim average in this case, at least, was worsened by Hindu performance in rural areas in general, by rural Hindu females in particular, and to some degree by rural Hindu males—in all of these categories, Hindu performance was worse than Muslim performance. Muslim males in general, too, did much better than their Hindu counterparts. This highlights why it is so important to dissect the data as much as possible, and look at more nuanced realities—and, accordingly, approaches to justice in general, and healthcare in particular. In the second case, STs did worse than SCs in all categories, except that urban female SCs were slightly worse off than their ST counterparts. Total national performance was better than both in all cases. We observe that while affirmative action policies were targeted at the STs as well, SCs have benefited much more than them, which seems to be reflected in their improvements in child survival over time across the surveys. Let us now consider their historical performance.

Tribe/Caste

Scheduled tribes are another traditionally disadvantaged group whose situation has worsened over time in terms of child survival. At the national level, they were doing better than not just the SCs (Figure 3.23), but also Muslims and Hindus until 1984 (Figure 3.24). All of them, especially Muslims and SCs, performed better than STs between 1984 and 1997, as a result of which STs did only slightly better than SCs, and substantially worse than others, by 1997. At the state level as well, with the exception of Andhra Pradesh in our selection—where they started out from being the worst to becoming the second best in 1984 and best by 1997—their situation has only worsened. In Rajasthan, they started out from being the best of all groups to becoming the worst by 1984,

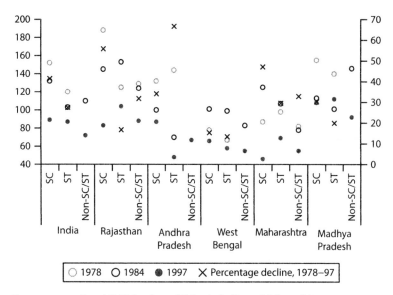

FIGURE **3.23** Rural IMR by Caste / Tribe in India and Selected States, 1978–97
Source: SRS.
Note: Circles map to the left axis, crosses to the right. Some data for non-SC / ST was not available.

and continued to be there subsequently. In West Bengal, from the best, they became fourth best in 1984 and third best by 1997. In Maharashtra, they started at the bottom, improved by a slot, then went to becoming the worst. In MP, from the second best, they became the best, and finally the worst. The broad overall pattern seems to be that of worsening situation over time. The case of females, tribals, and Muslims poses empirical challenges for the social determinants framework and normative challenges for several modern theories of justice.

SCs, however, fit perfectly within the standard discourse in social epidemiology—social status reflected in health status—as well as in health equity literature—marked, persistent inequalities between groups being inequitable and unjust. They were at the bottom of the caste hierarchy, where they remained on rural IMR too vis-à-vis others at the national level at least, between 1978 and 1997. The situation at the state level, however, was quite mixed. In Rajasthan, from the worst, they became the best, even including the Muslims. With the lowest rural IMR in 1984, and the highest per cent decline since 1978, a question

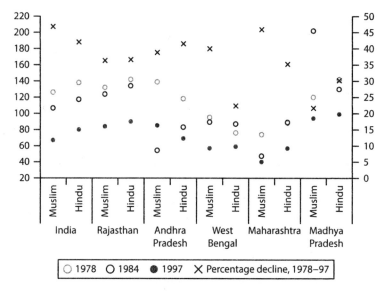

FIGURE 3.24   Rural IMR by Religion in India and Selected States, 1978–97
Source: SRS.
Note: Circles map to the left axis, crosses to the right. The circles for Hindu in Maharashtra almost overlap for years 1978 and 1984—the respective values are 88 and 89 respectively.

to be asked is—does child mortality in Rajasthan, thus, deserve least focus, or should we continue to go ahead with affirmative action based on historical injustice? Andhra Pradesh was also an exception for SCs, in a negative way though—unlike the STs, from the second best, their situation became the worst, both in terms of standing and percentage decline. In West Bengal too, they became the worst after 1978. In Maharashtra, from third, they became second best between 1978 and 1997, slipping down to the worst in 1984, despite the highest percentage decline. In MP, their journey was equally dramatic—from the worst, they became the second best and then the second worst by 1997, but with the highest per cent decline between 1978 and 1997. From the perspective of actual position, they would definitely merit policy focus, but this may not always be the case as far as improvement is concerned. The practice of justice has to be sensitive to both context and historical evolution.

Religion

The case of females, STs, and SCs was more or less straightforward, at least at the national level—for the former two, in terms of persistent worsening of the situation; for SCs, persistently remaining at/near the bottom. The case of Muslims, however, is quite complex, and as such the policy implications of their case would also be much more complex and interesting. If not the best, they were, in most cases, one of the best since the beginning and were able to either maintain or improve their position with a comparatively higher level of percentage decline.

At the national level, they started out as second only to STs and then by 1997, they emerged at the top with the highest percentage decline. In Rajasthan, while they managed to emerge at the top by 1984, they stood second to SCs in 1997 with a much lower percentage decline. Non-SC/STs did even worse—in such a situation, do we focus more on Muslims and non-SC/STs vis-à-vis the SCs/STs? In Andhra Pradesh, they started out worse than not just the Hindus generally, but also the SCs, but came out on the top in 1984, to slip down to the second worst slot in 1997. Variations between two time periods could also be due to some temporary, immediate factors during one of the time periods and we should, therefore, look at more time points to arrive at a stable analysis. West Bengal looks like a very interesting case—while STs had both the lowest percentage decline between 1978 and 1997 and lowest rural IMR in 1997, Muslims had the highest decline and the second worst position in 1997, from the worst in 1978. What do we do in such a situation? In Maharashtra, despite a slightly lower percentage decline than the SCs, Muslims continued to remain the best. In MP, they slipped from the best to the worst slot between 1978 and 1984, only to become the second best in 1997. There have been a lot of fluctuations, and we, thus, need to look at other as well as more recent, representative and reliable surveys.

Recent Data

Starting with survival in the first month (Figure 3.25), Muslims had the lowest NNMR during the NFHS-1 and NFHS-2 periods, but due to the lowest decline between NFHS-2 and NFHS-3, they had a slightly higher

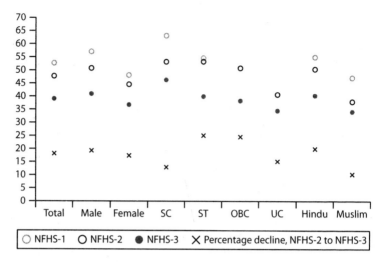

FIGURE 3.25   Neonatal Mortality Rate by Group, NFHS-1 to NFHS-3, India
Source: NFHS national reports.
Note: NFHS-1 did not present data for OBC and UC separately, hence not available in this and other figures. In such cases, therefore, we have presented the decline between NFHS-2 and NFHS-3.

rate than UCs in NFHS-3.[20] Despite a lower decline, females did better than males across all three surveys, highlighting persistence of biological advantage despite social disadvantage. Improvement in the case of STs was most dramatic between NFHS-2 and NFHS-3, though it was negligible between NFHS-1 and NFHS-2. Nevertheless, not only did they start out and end better than SCs, there seems to be a reversal in their fortune as far as these more recent surveys are concerned.

A similar picture emerges as far as Muslims and STs are concerned when we look at rural IMR (Figure 3.26), which we had considered in the previous special SRS surveys from 1978 to 1997. Muslims did the

[20] U5MR in NFHS-1 and NFHS-2 is for the 10-year period preceding the survey, while it is the five-year period for NFHS-3. This is not an issue as far as comparability is concerned, we just need to keep respective time periods in mind—1984–93 for NFHS-1, 1990–9 for NFHS-2 and 2002–6 for NFHS-3. Another clarification is that 'Other' in the caste category has been roughly taken to mean UCs. In NFHS-1, this category also included the OBCs, hence we did not include it here for comparison.

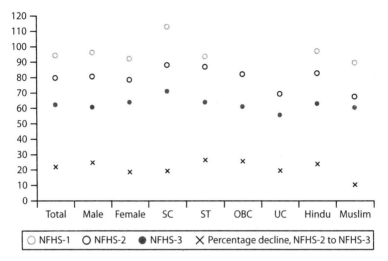

FIGURE 3.26   Rural IMR by Group, NFHS-1 to NFHS-3, India
Source: NFHS national reports.

best in NFHS-1 and NFHS-2, but with the lowest decline of all groups between NFHS-2 and NFHS-3, they fell considerably behind the UCs in NFHS-3. Hindus generally, with a much higher performance, closed the gap with Muslims, but still stayed slightly behind. STs, on the other hand, once again recorded the highest decline between NFHS-2 and NFHS-3, even as SCs, despite doing better during NFHS-1 and NFHS-2, continued to remain behind them across all three surveys. With a slower decline throughout, females, this time, eventually lost their advantage over males by NFHS-3. For females, the downward slide, in a relative sense, has continued, while it also started for Muslims at the national level, with the tide reversing in the case of STs.

The storyline does not change for Muslims even when we move on to survival in the first five years of birth (Figure 3.27), even as it worsens in the case of STs and females. Muslims were the best in NFHS-1 and only insignificantly behind UCs in NFHS-2 (U5MRs of 82.7 and 82.6 respectively), but due to the lowest decline between NFHS-2 and NFHS-3, they fell considerably behind the UCs as well as males on the whole, though they maintained, even if much smaller, lead over Hindus in NFHS-3. Females did worse than males and achieved a lower level of decline across all the three surveys, with their downward slide

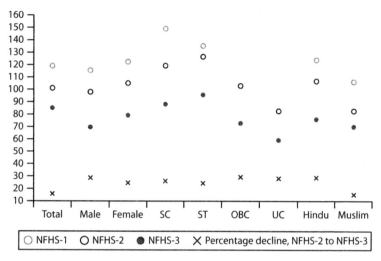

FIGURE 3.27   U5MR by Group, NFHS-1 to NFHS-3, India
Source: NFHS national reports.

continuing. STs started out much better vis-à-vis SCs, but with much lower decline between NFHS-1 and NFHS-2 ended up behind them in both NFHS-2 and NFHS-3. With almost no focus on social inequities in child survival in Indian policy, the fortunes of various groups have been left to fluctuate. Given the complexity of child survival in the country, I do not think anyone would argue in favour of a sense of (in)justice, let alone the current politics and practice of social justice. We discuss its policy and philosophical implications after discussing the access to determinants in the next chapter.

If outcomes are the ultimate decisive factor for priority-setting, highest policy focus on STs in the sphere of child survival does not seem to require much justification. However, what sort of interventions will be required in their case would be a complicated issue since, as we see in the next chapter, their journey from being the best to becoming the worst has *had* an inverse relationship with their access to modern healthcare. With low improvement over DHS surveys, the situation of females has only worsened, while in fact, they should be doing better than males due to their natural biological advantage, which makes their case even more deserving of policy attention. Equal standing with males would still be a disadvantage on their part—the biological

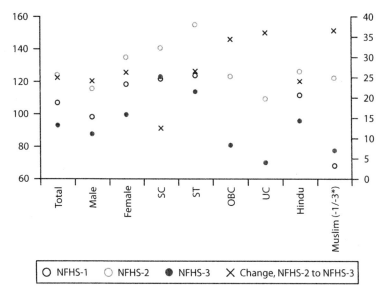

FIGURE 3.28   U5MR by Group, Rajasthan, NFHS-1 to NFHS-3
* Based on 250–499 unweighted cases.
Source: NFHS state reports.
Note: Circles map to the left axis, crosses to the right. The circles for SC almost overlap for NFHS-1 and NFHS-3—the respective values are 122 and 123 respectively.

optimal rather than social equality should be the deciding factor in their case. The situation of Muslims is complex as before—although they had one of the lowest U5MRs in NFHS-3, their percentage decline between NFHS-1 and NFHS-3 was only better than that of STs. The question to be asked here is—if STs and Muslims have had a historical advantage in child survival, which they have been losing in variable degrees over the years, do they merit policy focus to an extent that can enable them to regain their historical optimal?

At the state level (Figures 3.28 to 3.32), figures for NFHS-2 for all groups somehow increased vis-à-vis NFHS-1, particularly for Muslims. However, they experienced the highest decline between NFHS-2 and NFHS-3 in Rajasthan, and were only behind UCs in NFHS-3, while they were the best in NFHS-1 with a huge margin (as clarified earlier, UC data was not available for NFHS-1). SCs had the lowest decline and the highest U5MR in NFHS-3. Though STs were worse off than SCs, they stood better in NFHS-3, with a much higher decline. With much higher

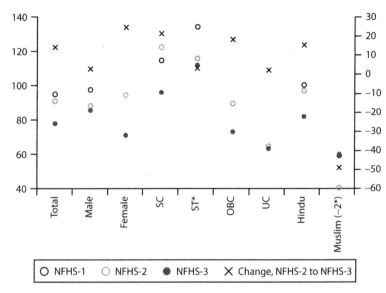

FIGURE 3.29   U5MR by Group, Andhra Pradesh, NFHS-1 to NFHS-3
* Based on 250–499 unweighted cases.
Source: NFHS state reports.
Note: Circles map to the left axis, crosses to the right. The circles for Female overlap for NFHS-1 and NFHS-2—the value was 95 for both. In the case of Muslim, they almost overlap for NFHS-1 and NFHS-3—the respective values were 59 and 60 respectively.

U5MR than males in NFHS-2, and a slightly higher decline, females were able to reduce the gender gap to some degree. In Andhra Pradesh, females experienced a much higher decline—the best of all—and ended up doing way better than males in NFHS-3. Muslims registered nearly 50 per cent decline between NFHS-1 and NFHS-2, but gained that much again between NFHS-2 and NFHS-3. They were followed by UCs with a decline of 2 per cent, and males and STs at 3 per cent. Despite lost fortunes, Muslims still had the lowest U5MR in all three surveys. India is quite a bewildering place not just in terms of its numerous cultures and dialects, but also vis-à-vis the understanding of inequities. What is a reasonable measure of justice in such a complex context?

In West Bengal, females started out worse than males, but with much higher declines between NFHS-1 and NFHS-2 as well as NFHS-2 and NFHS-3, they ended up having a much better U5MR. The situation of females seemed to have improved in NFHS surveys over the years in some of the selected states, and one must ask—should they still deserve

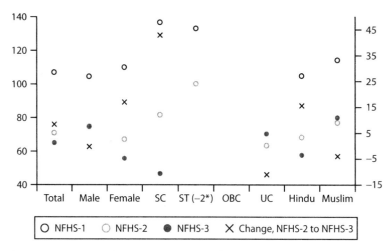

FIGURE **3.30**   U5MR by Group, West Bengal, NFHS-1 to NFHS-3
* Based on 250–499 unweighted cases.
Source: NFHS state reports.
Note: Circles map to the left axis, crosses to the right. OBC data was not available in any of the NFHS surveys. ST data for NFHS-3 and UC data for NFHS-1 was not available. The circles for Male overlap for NFHS-2 and NFHS-3—the value was 75 for both.

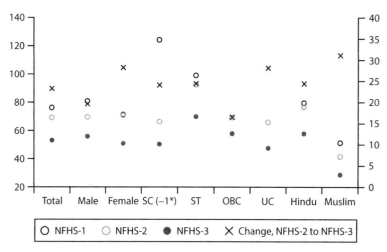

FIGURE **3.31**   U5MR by Group, Maharashtra, NFHS-1 to NFHS-3
* Based on 250–499 unweighted cases.
Source: NFHS state reports.
Note: Circles map to the left axis, crosses to the right. The circles for Female overlap for NFHS-1 and NFHS-2—the value was 71 for both.

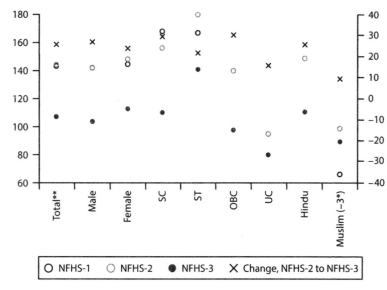

FIGURE 3.32   U5MR by Group, Madhya Pradesh, NFHS-1 to NFHS-3
* Based on 250–499 unweighted cases.
Source: NFHS state reports.
Note: Circles map to the left axis, crosses to the right. The circles for Total almost overlap for NFHS-1 and NFHS-2—the respective values were 143 and 144 respectively. The circles for Male overlap as well, with the value being 142. The circles for Hindu overlap for these two surveys with a value of 149.

more focus than males in these contexts? However, SCs were the star performers in this particular context, starting out as the worst and becoming the best by NFHS-3 with massive declines. The same question can be asked regarding them as well, especially vis-à-vis Muslims who had the worst U5MR in NFHS-3 as well as the UCs, who did better than SCs in NFHS-2, but with the worst decline (−11 per cent) fell even behind them, which is the first case of its kind in the entire country. Will we continue to focus on historical injustices against SCs even in a scenario where they have better outcome and improvement than the UCs?

In Maharashtra too, females did better than males between NFHS-2 and NFHS-3, and had lower U5MRs in both NFHS-1 and NFHS-3. Muslims had the highest level of decline and the lowest U5MR throughout. The SCs and UCs had equal U5MRs in NFHS-2, but with a slightly higher decline, the latter gained an edge by NFHS-3. With the exception of West Bengal, Muslims in all selected states as well as at the national level had a better U5MR than Hindus, though improvements between NFHS-2 and NFHS-3 in their case was only higher in Rajasthan and Maharashtra. In MP, females regularly had slightly higher U5MRs than males and also a slightly lower decline, which meant the gap increased by NFHS-3. But SCs, with the highest decline between NFHS-2 and NFHS-3, ended up having a much better U5MR than the STs and slightly better than females. Muslims had the lowest decline between NFHS-1 and NFHS-2 as well as NFHS-2 and NFHS-3, but still had the second lowest U5MR in NFHS-2 and NFHS-3, second to UCs only. The discussion of so many numbers might sound boring, but I have consciously brought them out here to demonstrate the bewildering complexity that the pursuit of justice has to deal with. Both the theorists and policymakers of justice appear naïve in the face of such complexity. The intention of this book is to enrich the philosophical and policy debates and pursuit of justice.

Let us close this section with a slightly deeper disaggregation of data. Figure 3.33 presents life expectancy at birth (LEB) by poverty,

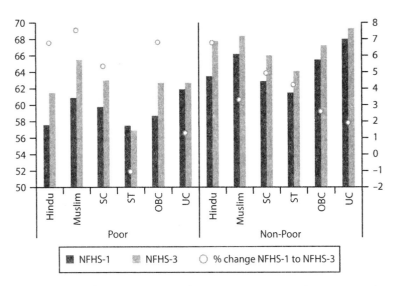

FIGURE 3.33   Life Expectancy at Birth (in Years) among Social Groups in India by Poverty
Source: IIPS 2010.
Note: Bars map to the left axis, circle to the right.

religion and caste/tribe for NFHS-1 and NFHS-3. STs had a lower LEB in the poor category during NFHS-3 than NFHS-1 with a decline in fortunes, while Muslims, with the highest performance, went to the top in NFHS-3, while starting out behind UCs in NFHS-1. In the non-poor category too, Hindus started and ended behind the Muslims despite a much higher improvement than the latter. STs improved slightly better than the Muslims, OBCs as well as UCs, but with a slightly lower improvement, they remained behind the SCs. Nevertheless, UCs started out and remained at the top, followed by Muslims in both NFHS-1 and NFHS-3.

Inter-State, Intra-Group Differentials

One of the ways in which we can analyse inter-state differentials is intra-group comparisons (Figures 3.34 to 3.41), by looking at how a particular group is doing or has done in different states. This will not only show their relative standing at the state level, but also their

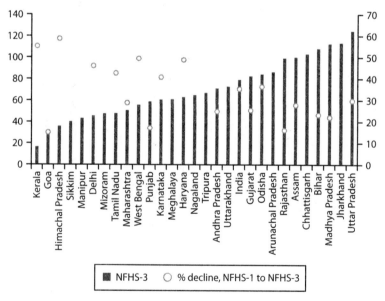

FIGURE 3.34   U5MR Differentials among Females, India and States/UTs, NFHS-1 to NFHS-3

Source: NFHS reports.

Note: Bars on the left axis, circle on the right.

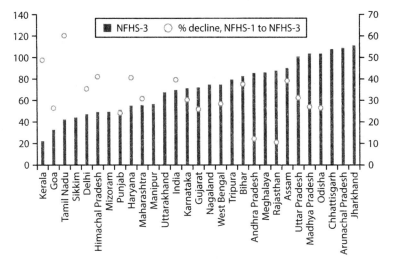

FIGURE 3.35   U5MR Differentials among Males, India and States/UTs,
NFHS-1 to NFHS-3
Source: NFHS reports.
Note: Bars on the left axis, circle on the right.

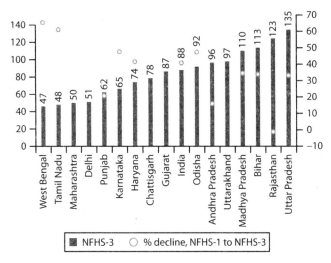

FIGURE 3.36   U5MR Differentials among Scheduled Castes, India and States/
UTs, NFHS-1 to NFHS-3
Source: NFHS reports.
Note: Bars on the left axis, circle on the right.

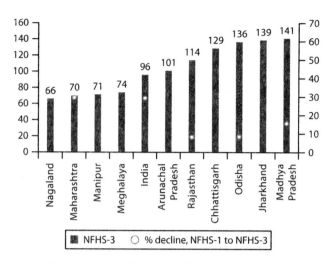

FIGURE 3.37   U5MR Differentials among Scheduled Tribes, India and States/
UTs, NFHS-1 to NFHS-3
Source: NFHS reports.
Note: Bars on the left axis, circle on the right.

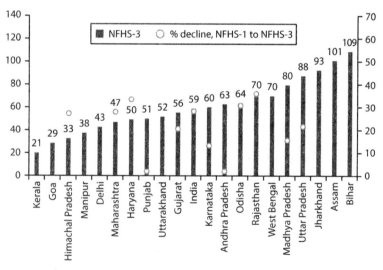

FIGURE 3.38   U5MR Differentials among Upper Castes, India and States/UTs,
NFHS-2 to NFHS-3
Source: NFHS reports.
Note: Bars on the left axis, circle on the right.

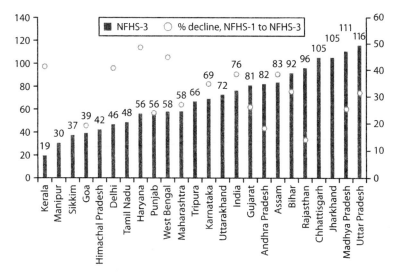

FIGURE **3.39** U5MR Differentials among Hindus, India and States/UTs, NFHS-1 to NFHS-3

Source: NFHS reports.

Note: Bars on the left axis, circle on the right.

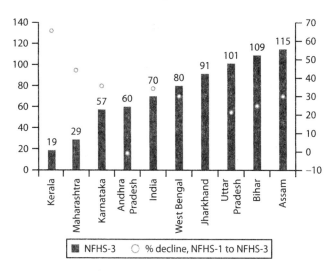

FIGURE **3.40** U5MR Differentials among Muslims, India and States/UTs, NFHS-1 to NFHS-3

Source: NFHS reports.

Note: Bars on the left axis, circle on the right.

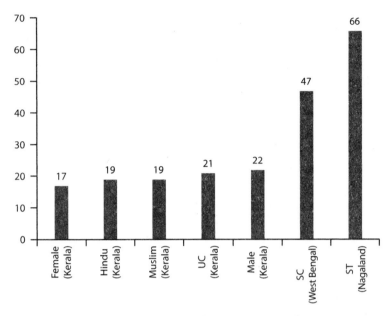

FIGURE **3.41**   Lowest U5MRs among Selected Groups in India, NFHS-3
Source: NFHS reports.

given maximal (if not the optimal) achievement in the country, and the shortfall in other states from their respective maximal. The maximals of various groups can be compared so that we can compare inter-group inequalities in the maximals along with inequalities in shortfalls and achievements vis-à-vis their respective maximals. The maximal of a group could be interpreted as the best that a particular group has been able to (empirically speaking)—not could potentially (normatively)—achieve in the given circumstances in the country. This is not an argument in favour of sociocultural essentialization, but rather against it—there are substantial variations among groups (defined by gender, caste, tribe, religion, and so on) that cannot be simplistically explained with reference to their sociocultural background *alone* and are the result of their specific contexts. It is not a mere coincidence that all groups had their maximals in Kerala—with the exception of SCs and STs, whose data from that state was not available (Figure 3.41). Kerala has not just had the best healthcare system in India for decades, but also land reforms as well as other favourable political economy factors.

Females there had a biological advantage over males, with Hindus and Muslims being equal. However, it was the reverse in SRS 2013 (see Figure 3.19).

Nevertheless, one could still argue that, in the given best of the health and social systems in the country, a particular group can achieve this much and its performance can be used as a yardstick for comparative purposes. If states can be compared with each other, why can't groups in them? This does not imply that we should ignore inter-group differentials at the intra-state levels, just that it might be worthwhile to make our evaluative base richer and more interesting. State-level policymakers can draw up lessons from other states in their effort to address group disparities or the general performance of particular groups in their own states. For example, policymakers in UP could learn how their counterparts in West Bengal and Tamil Nadu brought about major declines in child mortality among their respective Dalit populations (Figure 3.36).[21]

Figures 3.34 to 3.41 show how the selected groups have done across states. Differentials in female U5MR seem to be the most dramatic, ranging from 17 in Kerala to 125 in UP. The percentage decline in female U5MR over the years also varies dramatically—from 15 per cent in Goa to 59 per cent in Himachal Pradesh. The former, as per NFHS-3, had a female U5MR lower than that of the latter. A number of points can be quickly noted here. One, with this level of variation, it is difficult to generalize the situation of women in India, if child mortality is any indicator. Two, Kerala had the lowest U5MR as per NFHS-3 (19), and female U5MR in Kerala (17) was not just lower than the state average, but the lowest among any of the selected groups in the country (Figure 3.41). Therefore, it forms the lowest denominator, or the best possible in the country, from the perspective of which the performance of all others could potentially be assessed (that is, 'maximal average achievement' [Ruger 2009: 91]—we could also use a global maximal average achievement if we are concerned with global justice). However, we can argue that a female maximal average achievement can also be used for females

---

[21] See Mehdi (2014) for a discussion on why Dalits in UP have not been able to do good on this front despite decades of grassroots and political mobilization, and many years of rule by a Dalit Chief Minister (Mayawati of the Bahujan Samaj Party).

given their biological advantage in survival, and not for males, generally or across groups. Anyways, coming back to our discussion here, as per SRS 2013 (Figure 3.19), female U5MR in Kerala was higher than male U5MR, which matches with the national trend, making India stand behind even vis-à-vis the worst performers among the top five contributors to under five deaths worldwide, Pakistan and Nigeria—U5MR was 77 and 85 among females and males in Pakistan, 102 and 115 in Nigeria and 49 and 46 in India (2015).

As far as male U5MR is concerned, Kerala once again is the best state, Jharkhand the worst, with UP a few slots away from the worst. The highest percentage decline was in Tamil Nadu (60 per cent), the lowest in Rajasthan (11 per cent), between NFHS-1 and NFHS-3. Males in the laggard states of Bihar, Assam, and UP (UP had the worst U5MR in the country in the case of females) did better than those in Goa between NFHS-1 and NFHS-3, but Goan men were still way much better in terms of their NFHS-3 position.

As far as SCs are concerned, West Bengal experienced the highest decline and presently offers the lowest denominator in their case, followed by Tamil Nadu on both counts. Not surprisingly, therefore, Tamil Nadu did better overall as well. Despite decades of Dalit mobilization in the state, SC U5MR is the highest in UP, as for females. There is a lesson to be learnt in this regard from caste mobilization in Tamil Nadu (Mehrotra 2006). It is interesting to note that Rajasthan was once again one of the worst states, and in this particular case, the situation actually slightly worsened. STs too had a high lowest denominator (66 in Nagaland), with worst performance between NFHS-1 and NFHS-3, once again, being in Rajasthan. However, it was Maoist-concentration states of Jharkhand and MP which had the highest ST U5MRs in NFHS-3. Jharkhand was carved out of Bihar in the year 2000. In 1978, ST IMR in rural Bihar was 74, much better than not just the SCs (120), but the non-SC/ST population as well (88). In NFHS-3, ST IMR in Jharkhand was worst of all (93 vis-à-vis 77 among SCs and 76 among the UCs). Generally, progress on U5MR during NFHS surveys has been worst among them.

The aggregate situation affects everyone—some benefit more than others, some get less negatively affected than the others. Although UCs have generally done better than the SCs, with the exception of West Bengal in NFHS-3, and obviously than the STs, Figure 3.38

shows that there are vast differentials among UCs, in most cases linked to the overall performance of states—they do better in generally good-performing states, and worse in generally poor-performing states. Although we will discuss the conceptual implications of this at the end, let us quickly highlight two points here—(*a*) aggregate efficiency improvements are indispensable, and need to be considered along with equity considerations; (*b*) when aggregate situations are bad, we have to keep in mind the progress of all groups, not just that of the traditionally worse-off groups, since all of them get affected by a poor aggregate situation, even if differentially. Another interesting point as far as caste is concerned is that the OBCs in Kerala had better U5MR than the UCs there—13 and 21—and we can once again ask the question whether UCs, due to their traditional privilege, would deserve lesser policy focus.

From the perspective of two major religious groups in India—Hindus and Muslims—the lowest denominators are in Kerala (19). Muslims reached this value with a decline of 65 per cent between NFHS-1 and NFHS-3, Hindus with 42 per cent. They attained outcome equality with very different progress over time. The highest U5MR for Hindus in UP (116) is slightly higher than that of the Muslims in Assam (115).[22] With the exception of Muslim U5MR in Kerala, progress during NFHS surveys has not been spectacular for both groups in most states. The U5MR of Muslims in Andhra Pradesh actually worsened. In Maharashtra, despite some of the worst communal riots in recent Indian history, Muslims had their second best progress. Another notable thing is that the top three states for Muslims in terms of the NFHS-3 position also had the best progress over time. UP did worse than Bihar and Assam in the case of both Hindus and Muslims, but Muslim U5MR in UP was much lower (101) than that of Hindus. In NFHS-3, Muslim U5MR was worse than Hindu U5MR in only three states—West Bengal, Bihar, and Assam—as was the progress between NFHS-1 and NFHS-3, a clear case for focus on Muslims. Generally, however, why have Muslims had low

---

[22] Assam has had one of the highest percentages of Muslim population in the country, constituting 31 per cent of state population as per Census of India 2001. There have been several instances of riots against them in the state in the recent past.

U5MRs has been a matter of 'puzzle' and some explanations have been put forth, which we discuss in the next chapter. More importantly, we also discuss how we prioritize them based on the given data.

References

AHS. 2011. Press Release. 10 August. Available at http://pib.nic.in/newsite/PrintRelease.aspx?relid=74294 (accessed 5 August 2018).

Arokiasamy, P. 2007. 'Sex Ratio at Birth and Excess Female Child Mortality in India: Trends, Differentials and Regional Patterns'. In *Watering the Neighbours' Garden*, edited by Isabelle Attané and Christophe Guilmoto, 49–72. Paris: CICRED.

Arokiasamy, P. and A. Gautam. 2008. 'Neonatal Mortality in the Empowered Action Group States of India: Tends and Determinants'. *Journal of Biosocial Science* 40(2): 183–201.

CDS and UNFPA. 2009. 'Declining Child Sex Ratio (0–6 years) in India: A Review of Literature and Annotated Bibliography'. Data collected by Centre for Development Studies (CDS), Trivandrum, for United Nations Population Fund (UNFPA), India. https://india.unfpa.org/sites/default/files/pub-pdf/Declining%20CSR%20in%20India_%20Review%20of%20Literature%20and%20Annotated%20Bibloigraphy.pdf (accessed 5 August 2018).

Chandrasekhar, S. 1972. *Infant Mortality. Population Growth and Family Planning in India*. London: Allen & Unwin.

GoI. 2007. *Mortality Statistics in India 2006. Status of Mortality Statistics Reporting in India*. New Delhi: Central Bureau of Health Intelligence, Ministry of Health and Family Welfare (MoHFW), Government of India (GoI).

———. 2009. *Manual on Vital Statistics*. New Delhi: Central Statistical Organization (CSO), Ministry of Statistics and Programme Implementation (MoSPI), GoI.

Hill, Kenneth and Yoonjoung Choi. 2006. 'Neonatal Mortality in the Developing World'. *Demographic Research* 14(18): 429–52.

ICMR. 2007. *Health Research Policy—ICMR*. New Delhi: Indian Council of Medical Research.

IGME. 2015. *Levels and Trends in Child Mortality. Report 2015*. New York: Interagency Group for Child Mortality Estimation.

Jena, Binod Bihari, ed. 2012. 'Early Neonatal Mortality in India: A Study of Trends, Determinants and Inequalities'. Extended abstract submitted to Population Association of America 2012 Annual Meeting. Available at http://paa2012.princeton.edu/papers/120784 (accessed 5 August 2018).

Lawn, Joy E., Simon Cousens, and Jelka Zupan. 2005. '4 Million Neonatal Deaths: When? Where? Why?' *The Lancet* 365(9462): 891–900.

Lawn, J. E., K. Kerber, C. Enweronu-Laryea, and O. Massee Bateman. 2009. 'Newborn Survival in Low Resource Settings: Are We Delivering?' *BJOG: An International Journal of Obstetrics & Gynaecology* 116(s1): 49–59.

Mehdi, Ali. 2014. 'The Elusive Pursuit of Social Justice for Dalits in Uttar Pradesh'. In *Development Failure and Identity Politics in Uttar Pradesh*, edited by Roger Jeffery, Craig Jeffrey, and Jens Lerche, 75–103. New Delhi: SAGE.

Mehrotra, Santosh. 2006. 'Well-being and Caste in Uttar Pradesh: Why UP is not like Tamil Nadu'. *Economic and Political Weekly* 41(40): 4261–71.

Oestergaard, Mikkel Zahle, Mie Inoue, Sachiyo Yoshida, Wahyu Retno Mahanani et al. 2011. 'Neonatal Mortality Levels for 193 Countries in 2009 with Trends since 1990: A Systematic Analysis of Progress, Projections, and Priorities'. *PLoS Medicine* 8(8): e1001080: 1–13.

Padmadas, Sabu, Fiifi Johnson, Nyovani Madise, and Jane Falkingham. 2013. 'First-day Neonatal Mortality in the Developing World: A Neglected Crisis?'. Paper submitted to the XXV11 IUSSP International Population Conference, Busan, Korea (26–31 August 2013), Session 314: Health and Mortality in Childhood, Including Differences by Sex.

Pandey, Arvind, B.N. Bhattacharya, D. Sahu, and Rehana Sultana. 2005. 'Components of Under-five Mortality Trends, Current Stagnation and Future Forecasting Levels'. In *NCMH Background Papers*, edited by NCMH, 152–78. New Delhi: Ministry of Health & Family Welfare (MoHFW), GoI.

Ruger, Jennifer. 2009. *Health and Social Justice*. New York: Oxford University Press.

UNICEF. 2008a. *The State of the World's Children 2009. Maternal and Newborn Health*. New York: United Nations Children's Fund (UNICEF).

———. 2008b. *The State of Asia-Pacific's Children 2008. Child Survival*. New York: United Nations Children's Fund (UNICEF).

UNPD. 2015. *World Population Prospects 2015*. New York: Department of Economic and Social Affairs (DESA), Population Division.

WHO. 2006. *Neonatal and Perinatal Mortality. Country, Regional and Global Estimates*. Geneva: World Health Organization (WHO).

World Bank. 2004. *Attaining the Millennium Development Goals in India* (Report No. 30266-IN). New Delhi: Human Development Unit, South Asia Region, World Bank.

Zodpey, S. and V.K. Paul, eds. 2014. *State of India's Newborns 2014. A Report*. New Delhi: Public Health Foundation of India (PHFI), All India Institute of Medical Sciences (AIIMS) and Save the Children (SC).

4

The Architecture of Survival

A s discussed in Chapter 1, it is not too difficult to arrive at a consensus on child mortality as one of the top moral and policy concerns, which is reflected in several international covenants and development goals (MDG 4 and SDG 3.2). Saving children is a virtue by itself, and we do not need to have a justification for assigning top priority to it. That, however, cannot be said about the determinants of child survival. Despite the efforts of several highly prominent international organizations, policymakers, demographers, and others—not least the vaccination industry—to evolve an international consensus in favour of vaccinations as not just the elixir of life, but of life-long well-being and prosperity of children, their families, as well as the society at large,[1] the sphere of determinants is empirically,

[1] India's Union health and family welfare minister, Jagat Prakash Nadda, wrote a column in The Times of India ('So Our Children May Live', 28 April 2015), in which he mentioned how the government will promote vaccination, 'the best public health intervention', for all by 2020 under Mission Indradhanush. He goes on to generously conclude:

Known to be one of the most cost-effective interventions in the history of public health, vaccines do not merely save lives, they allow children and their families to thrive by preventing the onslaught of illness, disability, hospitalisation costs and needless human suffering. Vaccines also have long term benefits for individuals and society by contributing to improvements in cognitive development, educational attainment, labour productivity and economic development.

normatively as well as politically problematic, as this chapter would demonstrate.

A shift of focus from outcomes (child survival) to resources (determinants of child survival) also makes the pursuit of justice problematic, given that several aspects of parental (especially maternal) well-being are closely linked with children's survival, linking the pursuit of justice for children with a broader pursuit of justice. This is one of the reasons why well-intentioned organizations and individuals—such as the 'impatient optimists' (as Bill and Melinda Gates describe themselves)—who wish to save children without wasting any time have been trying hard to look for smart solutions like vaccines that can deliver quick and measurable results than wait for the slow and uncertain course of development and justice to make their mark. Their efforts have made a mark and saved the lives of millions of children around the world. However, the question remains—is bare survival the ultimate goal and to what degree can such quick-fix measures reduce the massive inequalities in which children are born and grow up?[2] At least, India's Union health minister seems quite *optimistic*,[3] although he does not sound *impatient* even as India continues to be the world's largest contributor to child deaths.

Let us begin with an overview of various determinants of child survival by broadly classifying them into three categories: (*a*) structural (political, economic, social structures); (*b*) intermediate (community, social/household status); and (*c*) immediate or biomedical (modern healthcare). We then look at available and comparable data on access to these determinants of health at the national and state levels, as well as among selected groups. Towards the end, we discuss whether the outcomes, as discussed in the previous chapter, resonate with access to these determinants. The policy and philosophical implications of this discussion are taken up in the following chapter.

[2] While fewer children are dying, the disability burden of child and maternal malnutrition in India has increased from more than 13 to 18 million years lived with disability (YLDs), according to estimates provided by the Global Burden of Disease, Institute for Health Metrics and Evaluation, Seattle (Washington), an institute which is also sponsored by the Gates Foundation. Bare survival is not enough for a country that aspires to overtake Great Britain by 2019 to become the world's fifth largest economy. See 'India Poised to Pip Britain to Become 5th Largest Economy Next Year: Arun Jaitley', *Times of India*, 13 July 2018.

[3] See n 1.

Structural Determinants

The Michael Marmot-led Commission on Social Determinants of Health (CSDH), established by the WHO in 2005, made an attempt to normatively recast the increasingly sterile and techno-managerial debates on child mortality by arguing that it is not lack of biomedical healthcare, but 'a toxic combination of poor social policies, unfair economics, and bad politics' which has been responsible for premature deaths, poor health and 'much of health inequity', and 'the main action on social determinants of health must therefore come from outside the health sector' (CSDH 2008). This resonates with constant references to multisectorality in the discussion of health-related SDGs. A typical social determinants approach (SDA) argues that socio-economic and political structures (global, national, local) influence our social position, which impacts our material circumstances, biological and behavioural factors, access to healthcare, and eventually, our chances of survival, health, and well-being (Figure 4.1). From CSDH's perspective, 'why treat people ... then send them back to the conditions that made them sick?' (CSDH 2008). The root, the structural determinants, have to be addressed if subsequent interventions, especially at the biomedical level, have to produce meaningful results.

Inasmuch as it builds on the work of social epidemiologists—who have focused on meso-level neighbourhood, community, and class

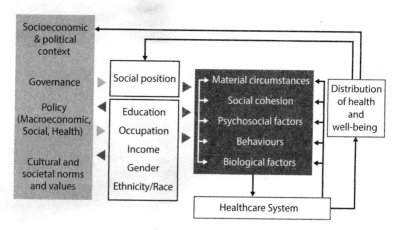

FIGURE 4.1   Conceptual Framework of the CSDH
Source: CSDH (2008: 43).

factors since the early nineteenth century—this narrative does not have much new to offer, although it did bring about a renewed focus on the SDA. However, what makes it distinct—albeit not without any precedent—is its focus on *political epidemiology*, a new area of study which focuses on the role of macro-level political structures, institutions, and policies and their impact on not just our social, but also health, status, and inequalities.[4] Among the pioneers of this area of research has been Vicente Navarro, whose work has focused on the health impact of political parties in power. In one of the papers, Navarro and Shi (2001), argue—with some qualifications obviously, given that this is still an under-investigated field—that political parties, in power for longer periods, committed to socio-economic redistributive policies, have generally been successful in reducing social inequities and, thereby, health outcomes like child mortality. In the Indian context, Navarro and Shi (2001) pointed out that while the impressive health achievements of Kerala have been widely studied, only few studies have linked them with its political context. Although they did not refer to it as one of these few, Ratcliffe (1977) had argued earlier that Kerala's political economy played a role in its mortality and fertility achievements. Navarro (2000: 661) also criticized Amartya Sen's approach to development for the 'absence of an analysis of the power relations that cause and reproduce underdevelopment through national and international political institutions'. One can argue that Sen's approach to development was more normative rather than empirical, and so it did not focus too much on the myriad challenges to development—power relations being one of them, although powerful.

Talking about the role of governments towards the right to health, a WHO factsheet argues that 'governments must generate conditions in which everyone can be as healthy as possible. Such conditions range from ensuring availability of health services, healthy and safe working conditions, adequate housing and nutritious food.'[5] However, another WHO report argues that 'a common misconception is that the State has to guarantee us good health. However, good health is influenced by several factors that are outside the direct control of States, such as

---

[4] For some background on this, see Pega et al. (2013).

[5] The right to health (WHO Factsheet No. 323, November 2013). See http://www.who.int/mediacentre/factsheets/fs323/en/ (accessed 23 May 2015).

an individual's biological make-up and socio-economic conditions' (OHCHR and WHO 2008: 5). It is surprising that 'socio-economic conditions' are seen as 'outside the direct control of States', although one might agree that 'good health' cannot always be guaranteed. Nevertheless, what is problematic is that we do not yet have a clear delineation of the responsibility of the State—and by implication, of others—regarding whatever is guaranteed under the right to life or health. This is one area of concern where the engagement of political philosophy and political economy in public health debates is clearly vindicated. Epidemiologists can inform these debates through their understandings of pathways, but cannot convincingly argue about the appropriate role of the State in public health. This discussion is intrinsically normative, and that is the element that the CSDH has tried to re-infuse in existing debates on health in general, premature mortality in particular. Health and survival are intrinsically a normative concern, and cannot be left entirely to policy technocrats, doctors, epidemiologists, pharma companies, philanthropists, and the like.

Another, and probably the most important, dimension of structural determinants is the role of the economy—inasmuch as it determines our ability to access not just the medical, but also the social determinants of health, especially in situations where the role of the State is limited due to principle, paucity of resources, inefficiency, corruption, or any other factor. We could refer to it as *economic epidemiology*—a focus on the influence of economic structures, institutions and processes on access to broader resources for health and health outcomes—but not in the conventional use of the term—that is, economic incentives or 'nudge' for adopting individual healthy behaviours. From a Marxist perspective, economy is the base on which the superstructure of political, social, health, and other systems are built, and scholars in this school have argued about health access and outcomes being sensitive to the nature of the predominant economy at the global and national levels. From their perspective, even a relatively poor state based on principles of a socialist economy is able to achieve health outcomes comparable to or better than a rich state based on the principles of a free market economy—by virtue of the former being predominantly involved in people's health as well as other spheres of social development. We know how this has worked in the case of Kerala, but not in the case of West Bengal, in the Indian context. At an international level, Cuba, with a GDP per capita slightly more than 10 per cent of the United States (USD 6,051 and USD 49,804 respectively), and health expenditure per capita (current USD) much less than 10 per cent (USD 648 and USD 8,553 respectively), had a better U5MR than the latter (6.9 and 7.2 respectively) in 2011 (WDI). At the same time, these examples reflect how political commitment matters more than resources for health outcomes—probably more so than the economic epidemiological one from a Marxist perspective.

Anyway, the CSDH has tried to combine not just the social and political, but also the economic strand of epidemiology into its framework to produce a discourse which is being acknowledged worldwide, but not necessarily being acted upon in its broadest sense, given the sensitivities of the status quo and, not least, the way government departments are generally structured, posing a challenge to coherent multisectoral action on the social determinants of health. Like theories of justice, operationalization is the key challenge here too. Instead, the bar of outcome has been lowered to minimally affect the status quo—the socio-economic, political, and the governmental. At the same time, one could argue that the CSDH is as bold as international organizations like the WHO—dependent on funding from member states—can get in their officially stated capacities, and have to be content with 'tame' goals such as the MDGs and SDGs in the name of global justice. I do not wish to undermine the significance of such goals for international development in some of the most fundamental areas of continuing deprivation around the world. However, I feel that they are not sufficient in the context of global injustices and tend to wean our attention away from the larger issues by keeping us preoccupied with the basic. Independent academics should adopt an increasingly interdisciplinary and normative approach, invoking theories of justice in a rigorous and sustained manner to address challenges of public health. Non-communicable diseases (NCDs) are an emerging area of concern where such an approach would be of great help, given that broader determinants are already widely recognized in their case. However, at the same time, there are efforts to shift the focus towards individual behavioural determinants by governments to escape their share of blame and responsibility, and towards diagnosis and treatment by pharmaceutical firms in order to expand their customer base with new entrants as well as enhancements in survival prospects of those already within the fold. A broader diagnosis—and treatment—are urgently required.

Intermediate Determinants

The sphere of intermediate determinants is what most social epidemiological studies have focused on. Marmot himself had led another team for the famous Whitehall studies, conducted between 1967 and 1988, that identified a persistent 'social class gradient' in health even among British civil servants. Contemporaneously, Douglas Black and his team highlighted 'marked inequalities in health between the social classes in Britain' in their well-known *Black Report* of 1980. In Britain itself, more than a century earlier, vast differences in life expectancy across occupational groups were reported by Edwin Chadwick in his 'Report on the sanitary condition of the labouring population and on the means of its improvement' (1842), which became the basis for Britain's first Public Health Act in 1848. Around that time, in 1844, Friedrich Engels had provided 'evidence regarding higher mortality among poor houses in poor compared to 'improved' streets' in 'The condition of the working class in England' (Krieger 2011). Even a few decades earlier, between 1820 and 1830, Louis-René Villermé, the French physician and early pioneer of social epidemiology, conducted a series of studies, highlighting correlations between death rates among prisoners and their detention conditions as well as the patterning of mortality rates across Parisian neighbourhoods by poverty and wealth (Julia and Valleron 2011; Krieger 2011). Similar evidence is also available from a number of other developed countries.[6]

Thanks to DHS and other surveys, we also have recent evidence on the role of socio-economic variables like maternal education and household wealth on child survival from the developing world as well.[7] Figures 4.2 and 4.3 show IMR differentials in DHS 2005/06 surveys by maternal education and household wealth. Education and economic status are interlinked to a degree—wealthy people tend to be educated,

---

[6] See, for instance, Guralnick (1963); Kitagawa and Hauser (1973); Kunst (1997); Navarro (1990); Nelson (1992); van der Heyden et al. (2009); Wilkinson (1989).

[7] For example, refer to Bicego and Ties Boerma (1993) for data from 17 developing countries; Caldwell (1979) for analysis with reference to Nigerian data; Caldwell and McDonald (1982) for data from the World Fertility Survey on 10 third world countries; and Schell et al. (2007) for a study of 152 low, middle, and high income countries.

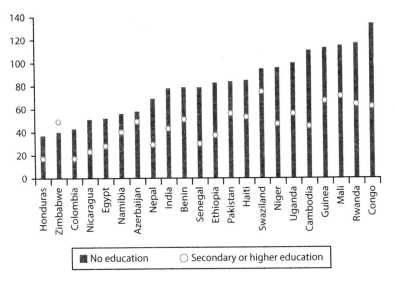

FIGURE 4.2   IMR in DHS Countries by Level of Maternal Education, 2005 / 2006
Source: DHS.

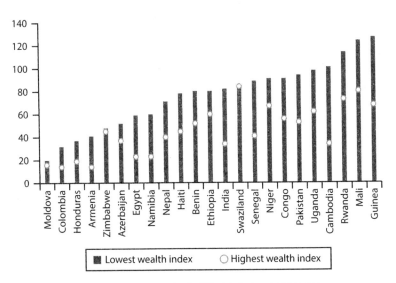

FIGURE 4.3   IMR in DHS Countries by Wealth Index, 2005 / 2006
Source: DHS.

educated people tend to be wealthy. Nevertheless, in the case of child survival, both factors tend to have a 'strong, independent effect' (Rutstein and Johnson 2004). In other words, even the educated poor or the rich uneducated would have relatively better child survival prospects vis-à-vis their less fortunate peers—one of the neglected benefits of education.

Before moving further, let us briefly discuss the notion of 'structural violence' or 'structural discrimination'. Although these terms give the impression that they should be part of structural determinants, they actually focus on social discrimination and its negative impact on economic as well as health status (Figure 4.4). Farmer, Commons, and Simmons (1996: 369) defined structural violence as 'a series of large-scale forces—ranging from gender inequality and racism to poverty—which structure unequal access to goods and services'. While Gilligan (1997: 192) saw it, in a more direct sense from a health perspective, as the 'increased rates of death and disability suffered by those who occupy the bottom rungs of society, as contrasted with the relatively lower death rates experienced by those who are above them'. These notions are quite helpful when we wish to explain pathways through

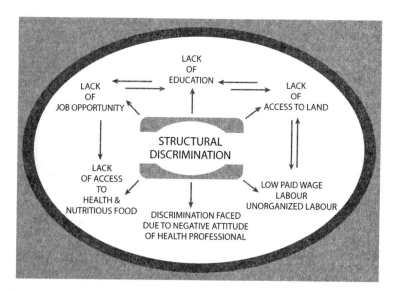

FIGURE 4.4   Impact of Structural Discrimination
Source: Chatterjee and Sheoran (2007: 6).

which variables in social epidemiological studies affect our access to wealth and health status. The lack of explanation of such mechanisms has been what Mosley and Chen (1984) have referred as the 'black box' in social scientific understanding of health. We discuss how they tried to address these lacunae through their model of child survival, health, and nutrition in the next section. Before we move on, let me quickly state that the distinction between various levels of determinants, especially the structural and the intermediate, is not watertight, with several over-laps and inter-linkages between them, some of which we refer to in the section after the next.

Immediate Determinants

The shift in focus towards neonatal mortality, as discussed in the previous chapter, also appears to be a shift of sorts towards the immediate, more biomedical and individual determinants of child survival such as antenatal care (ANC),[8] postnatal care (PNC),[9] institutional deliveries, vaccinations, and so on. According to the UN's Inter-agency Group for Child Mortality Estimation (IGME), 'neonatal mortality ... is of interest because the health interventions needed to address the major causes of neonatal deaths generally differ from those needed to address other under-five deaths' (IGME 2011: 9). Figure 4.5 shows variations in IMR in 2005/06 DHS surveys by antenatal and delivery care, which are

---

[8] Antenatal care is 'care provided by skilled health-care professionals to pregnant women and adolescent girls in order to ensure the best health conditions for both mother and baby during pregnancy. The components of ANC include: risk identification; prevention and management of pregnancy-related or concurrent diseases; and health education and health promotion' (WHO 2016: 1). At least three ANC check-ups are to be provided to pregnant women under India's RCH programme.

[9] Postnatal care is provided soon after delivery to protect the health of the mother and the newborn child, especially when deliveries take place in non-institutional settings. Like ANC, three PNC check-ups are recommended under RCH. The WHO defines the postnatal period as the first six weeks after birth, considered as 'critical to the health and survival of a mother and her newborn'. See www.who.int/pmnch/media/publications/aonsectionIII_4.pdf (accessed 29 December 2017).

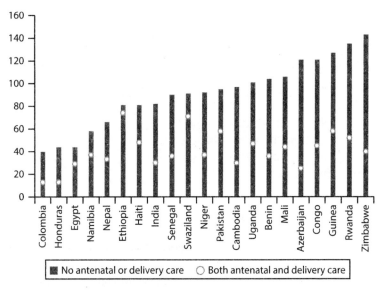

FIGURE 4.5 IMR in DHS Countries by Antenatal and Delivery Care, 2005/2006
Source: DHS.

much dramatic than variations by education level or wealth, especially in Azerbaijan, Zimbabwe, Honduras, Cambodia, and Colombia.

It has been argued that cost-effective maternal and newborn care can address the determinants of neonatal mortality.[10] According to the Agha Khan Development Network (AKDN), children in South Asia 'do not survive because of parental ignorance or because communities in remote regions do not have access to affordable and effective lifesaving interventions such as oral rehydration solution (ORS) for diarrhoea, antibiotics to treat respiratory infections, and antimalarial tablets'.[11] WHO claims to have a 'mother–baby package' (Integrated Management of Pregnancy and Childbirth or IMPAC) that costs USD 3

[10] See Arokiasamy and Gautam (2008); Bhalotra, Valente, and van Soest (2010); Darmstadt et al. (2005); Pradhan and Arokiasamy (2010); The Million Death Study Collaborators (2010); Wardlaw et al. (2014).

[11] 'Child Survival Programme', http://www.akdn.org/india_survival.asp (accessed 23 May 2012).

a year per capita and includes ANC, PNC, normal delivery care assisted by a skilled birth attendant, family planning advice, and the management of sexually transmitted infections not only to save maternal and infant deaths, but also to prevent life-long disability due to complications during pregnancy and childbirth.[12]

Primary health systems in developing countries would have to be strengthened if they are to address the immediate determinants of child survival, that too in a reductionist sense, with other related sectors exonerated from their respective roles toward child survival. I am reminded of a Persian couplet, whose author I am not able to recall—*'aasman baar-i amanat ra na-tawanist kasheed, qura-i faal be naam-i man-i deewane zadand'* ('heavens could not bear the burden of the Trust [freedom/choice], the dice of fate fell in my stupid's name').[13] However, 'defining development down', a phrase used regarding the 'low, limited and specific' nature of the MDGs (Pritchett and Kenny 2013), there has been an effort to even forego systemic change at a primary health level, not to talk of higher-order structural and intermediate determinants, and further limit the focus to one or two most important interventions assumed to be most straightforward and effective in substantially reducing child mortality and improving life prospects, those that could be delivered to the target groups at their doorstep. Consider the following statements from WHO:

> For some of the most deadly childhood diseases, such as measles, vaccines are available and timely completion of immunization protects a child from this illness and death.... About 20 million young children worldwide are severely malnourished, which leaves them more vulnerable to illness and early death.... Around three quarters of malnourished children can be treated with 'ready-to-use therapeutic foods'.[14]

[12] 'Health, a Key to Prosperity: Success Stories in Developing Countries', http://www.who.int/inf-new/mate.htm (accessed 21 May 2012).

[13] This is inspired by the Quranic verse 72, chapter 33—'We did indeed offer the Trust to the heavens and the earth and the mountains; but they refused to undertake it, being afraid thereof: but man undertook it; surely, he is unjust, ignorant.' From our perspective, primary health systems are expected to deliver what higher-order systems have not been able to deliver in the Indian context— child survival and health.

[14] 'Child Mortality', http://www.who.int/maternal_child_adolescent/topics/ child/mortality/en/ (accessed 23 May 2015).

In Bangladesh, one of the world's least developed countries, over 80% of women give birth without any help from a skilled birth attendant. Most deliveries take place at home, often in conditions of very poor hygiene—placing the lives of both mother and child at risk.... Yet despite this unpromising start to life, death rates for neonatal tetanus in newborn babies have been reduced by over 90% in Bangladesh in little more than a decade. The turnaround is the result of mass immunization campaigns to protect women of childbearing age against tetanus infection. Nationwide efforts to increase coverage with tetanus toxoid vaccine have boosted immunization rates from 5% in 1986 to 86% by 1998.[15]

If deadly childhood diseases and risk factors could be so effectively addressed through cheap vaccinations—the pentavalent vaccine, for example, is said to protect children against five life-threatening diseases and is now being offered at an average price of 84 US cents per dose[16]—and child malnutrition 'treated' with therapeutic foods, without deliveries being attended by skilled health personnel (without reform of primary health systems) or without proper hygiene at home (without reforming public health systems or addressing intermediate or structural factors), why bother about institutional reforms even at the immediate level? For UNICEF, 'vaccines are by far our most important commodities'.[17] All we need to do is to identify those who are deprived of vaccinations and reach out to them. Bill Gates, during an interview with CNN, talked about sense of justice and the inequity in access to vaccines between rich and poor kids, presenting vaccines as the be-all and the end-all of child survival.[18] This approach is not new (for example, see Mosley and Becker 1991). Nevertheless, barring the few who do not acknowledge the role of structural and intermediate determinants of survival and health, most other representatives of this framework decide to focus on the immediate determinants largely due to pragmatic empirical

[15] 'Health, a Key to Prosperity'.

[16] UNICEF Press Release, 'Supply of children's five-in-one vaccine secured at lowest-ever price' (Geneva, 19 October 2016), https://www.unicef.org/media/media_92936.html (accessed 26 December 2017).

[17] UNICEF Supply Division Deputy Director, Stephen Jarrett, 'A global leader in vaccine supply'. http://www.unicef.org/immunization/index_leader.html (accessed 21 May 2012).

[18] Justifying his pledging of USD 10 billion to provide vaccinations to children around the world over the next decade, Gates argued: 'Over this decade,

or normative considerations. Linkages of immediate determinants with survival and health are straightforward and understandable for policy-makers, donors, and the public alike, and they can be made relatively easily and cheaply available—and most importantly, without disturb-ing the political, social, and economic status quo. During interviews I conducted in 2009 in New Delhi, several international organizations acknowledged the role of structural and intermediate determinants,[19] but argued they have to be cautious, lest they hurt the sensitivities of the host nations and be asked to leave. The pursuit of justice pertains to all levels of determinants, but is confronted by a reductionist, minimal-ist tendency on the one hand, and a resourcist one on the other. Both tendencies need to be resisted in the pursuit of justice and health.

Interlinkages between Determinants

The three layers of determinants of survival and health are linked with each other in simple as well as complex ways. Structural determi-nants, in many a case, influence access to intermediate determinants. Intermediate determinants, in their turn, especially in countries with deficient or discriminatory public health systems, not only influence access to the immediate determinants as well as to other intermedi-ate determinants of child survival like nutrition and neighbourhood, they also affect patterns at the structural level—for instance, socially

---

we believe unbelievable progress can be made, in both inventing new vaccines and making sure they get out to all the children who need them. We could cut the number of children who die every year from about 9 million to half of that, if we have success on it. We have to do three things in parallel: Eradicate the few that fit that profile—ringworm and polio; get the coverage up for the vaccines we have; and then invent the vaccines—and we only need about six or seven more—and then you would have all the tools to reduce childhood death, reduce population growth, and everything—the stability, the environment ...'. See http://edition.cnn.com/2011/HEALTH/02/03/gupta.gates.vaccines.world. health/ (accessed 24 May 2015).

[19] Consider two tweets, for instance, which reflect their concern for the larger determinants of health and survival—'Gender equality must remain top priority to close health equity gap' (@UN_Women, UN Women, 19 May 2015); 'Maternal mortality is in part a manifestation of various forms of discrimination against women' (@USAIDGH, USAID Global Health, 20 May 2015).

dominant groups like the upper castes also dominate the polity and economy to a substantial level. On the other hand, at the structural level, if there is a strong political commitment to healthcare, even if the economic and social systems are inequitable, it may lead to a liberal public financing/universal provision of the immediate determinants of health, making the structural and the intermediate economic variables less influential as far as access to immediate determinants are concerned. According to Wardlaw et al. (2014: 2–3), 'substantial progress in some countries demonstrates that combining political commitment, sound strategies and adequate resource makes it possible to rapidly reduce neonatal mortality, regardless of national income'. Political commitment, especially for health in developing nations, usually arises as a result of grassroots mobilization, which, in turn, is influenced by political, economic and social structures. Nag (1983) attributed Kerala's health achievements to its higher social development—mass mobilization led to extensive public provision of healthcare and education, which, in turn, led to higher utilization of healthcare. Political and social repression as well as economic vulnerability limit the space for such mobilization, and in such contexts, public provision or financing of healthcare is usually low. Nevertheless, even with public financing or universal provision, the utilization of immediate determinants may still be dependent on community,[20] parental, especially maternal, education[21] (the intermediate education variable). And even if healthcare utilization is high and equitable, the socio-economic gradient in health and survival would still persist—though in muted forms—as access to the level and quality of healthcare as well as other determinants

[20] If an educated person lives in an uneducated community, the neighbourhood effect might tend to neutralize the potential benefits of that person's education for his or his family's health. Similarly, in households where household elders or fathers are predominant, maternal education will not be able to play a *decisive* role as far as decisions about their own or children's health is concerned. In such societies, the educational level of at least both parents, if not that of household elders, should also be taken into consideration.

[21] 'Schooling makes parents increasingly part of a new culture—a global culture of largely Western origin.… [C]hildren (and women) are awarded higher priorities in terms of care and consumption than in the traditional system' (Caldwell and McDonald 1982: 266).

would still be dependent on socio-economic status (for example, the social gradient among Whitehall bureaucrats). In any case, we have to keep in mind that there are outliers to discussed pathways and determinants—given alternative systems of healthcare and other factors—that continue to baffle those who stick to them dogmatically. STs and Muslims in India are cases in point.

However, even for neonatal mortality, addressing at least some of the structural or intermediate determinants will be critical. If we look at major causes of neonatal deaths in India (Figure 4.6), at least the two top ones, accounting for 63 per cent of such deaths, are linked to household and institutional care of mother and child than to vaccinations. Preterm births is the largest killer—India again leading the list with more than three times more preterm births than China on the second spot. According to WHO, 'to reduce preterm birth rates, women need better access to family planning and increased empowerment, as well as improved care before, between and during pregnancies'.[22] 'Increased empowerment' of women is related with the structural and intermediate determinants, as is their access to 'improved care' in several instances. Studies on the determinants of neonatal deaths have emphasized the role of these larger determinants, and even that of the

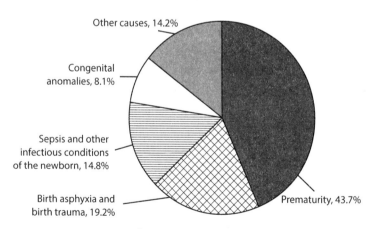

FIGURE 4.6   Major Causes of Neonatal Deaths (0–27 Days), India, 2013
Source: WHO.

[22] 'Preterm birth', http://www.who.int/mediacentre/factsheets/fs363/en/ (accessed 24 May 2015).

underlying cultural causes of death, for many of the immediate clinical causes of death.[23]

Chattopadhyay et al. (2004: 2–3) argue that 'education, religion and work status of the mother have significant effects' even on early neonatal mortality 'besides the so-called biological and health care factors'. For Lawn, Cousens, and Zupan (2005: 895), 'poverty is an underlying cause of many neonatal deaths, either through increasing the prevalence of risk factors such as maternal infection, or through reducing access to effective care'. Talking in the context of 'starvation deaths' in Bengal during 1943–6, Sen (2012: 203) argued that conventional categories of causes of death do not typically include such causes as starvation, even though 'it is common to die of starvation through diarrhoea', which was the third largest cause of death in rural as well as urban India among under-one children (RGI 2009). Figure 4.7 shows that undernutrition is the underlying cause of several immediate causes of child deaths. Official causes of death in India are medically certified, which means they are restricted to immediate biomedical factors, which is perfectly fine. However, medical certifications do not mean higher determinants do not exist.

Mosley and Chen (1984), through their model of child health and survival (Figure 4.8), regarded a classic in public health literature, tried to bridge the gap between disparate understandings of intermediate (social scientific) and immediate (medical) determinants.[24] From their viewpoint, 'all social and economic determinants must operate through these [that is, proximate] variables to affect child survival' (1984: 27). In their model, the 'must operate' condition seems justified, though the way we have outlined these determinants above, intermediate determinants do not operate only through immediate determinants, but directly too. Nevertheless, what is important is 'the need for a multidisciplinary approach to understanding and alleviating child mortality … child mortality should be studied more as a chronic disease process with multifactorial origins than as an acute, single-cause phenomenon' (1984: 40–1). Many a time, it is lack of such an understanding of

---

[23] Black, Morris, and Bryce (2003); Lawn, Cousens, and Zupan (2005); WHO (2006).

[24] For them, intermediate or proximate determinants are the ones in grey boxes in the figure.

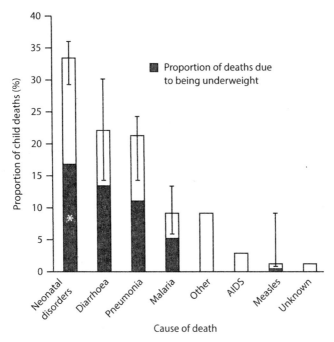

FIGURE 4.7   Proportion of Immediate Causes of Child Deaths Due to Being Underweight
*Implies work in progress to establish cause-specific contribution of being underweight to neonatal deaths.
Source: Black, Morris, and Bryce (2003: 2230).

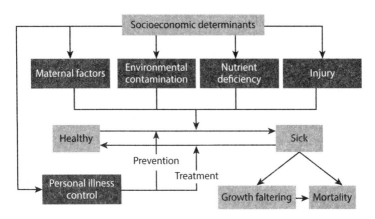

FIGURE 4.8   Determinants of Child Health and Survival
Source: Mosley and Chen (1984: 29).

pathways of child survival or mortality which leads to confusion and reductionist claims by the advocates of both socio-economic/political and biomedical factors. Both upstream and downstream factors have to be taken into consideration for a comprehensive understanding of the determinants of survival.

Contextual Nature of Determinants

Black, Morris, and Bryce (2003) have argued that causes of child deaths 'differ substantially' across countries. That could be the case even within countries, particularly if they are as large and diverse as India. According to the Million Death Study, 'five avoidable causes accounted for nearly 1.5 million child deaths in India in 2005, with substantial differences between regions and sexes' (The Million Death Study Collaborators 2010: 1853). One could argue the same for groups—as we see further—within and across countries as well as individuals within them. Figures 4.2, 4.3, and 4.5 highlight the intra-country differentials in IMR by maternal education (1), wealth index (2) and antenatal and delivery care (3), and also show their differential impact at the inter-country level. In Zimbabwe, for instance, quite unexpectedly, mothers with secondary or higher education recorded a higher IMR vis-à-vis those with no education,[25] negligible differential between those in the highest and lowest wealth indices, while IMR among mothers with no antenatal or delivery care was the highest in the selection. Elsewhere, mothers with no education had an IMR which was 18 (Azerbaijan) to 163 (Senegal) percentage higher vis-à-vis mothers with secondary or higher education—with India standing in the middle at 81 per cent. As far as the wealth index was concerned, this variation ranged from 0 per cent (Swaziland) to 197 per cent (Cambodia)—with India towards the higher end of the spectrum at 141 per cent higher IMR among those in the lowest wealth index in comparison to those in the highest. Differentials by antenatal and delivery care were the highest, ranging from 9 per cent in Ethiopia to 384 per cent in Azerbaijan—with India standing at 173 per cent. Equality of opportunities (determinants), anyone?

---

[25] Kembo and van Ginneken (2009) point out that the 1994 and 1999 DHS surveys in Zimbabwe showed a larger impact of maternal education on infant mortality than the 2005–6 survey, whose data is presented here.

Contextuality adds to the complexity of determinants in a major way. What we had discussed in the previous section was expected influences and pathways through which determinants lead to outcomes. However, their actual impact varies dramatically by context, as do pathways of influence, necessitating localized/contextually-sensitive interventions to address child mortality. We had mentioned in the second chapter, in a conceptual frame though, that pervasive human diversity in internal and external characteristics means that people need different quantities of the same or even different sets of resources to achieve similar outcomes. For instance, even if two groups/individuals had similar levels of child mortality and resided in the same locality, there would at least be some peculiar determinants of mortality and, accordingly, at least a slightly varied set of interventions for survival needed. Then, there is the issue of choice which those considered responsible for children should have in the selection of interventions—requiring a reasonably plausible plurality of interventions to be made available to them if they are to be held responsible.

Even if there are asymmetries of information in healthcare, a certain type of healthcare or intervention (no matter how 'scientific') cannot be forced on an individual or group just because 'experts' assume it to be the best for them—or for everyone around the world. The controversy around vaccinations among Muslims in South Asia is a case in point. Although it seems like a normative rather than an empirical issue, along with empirical human diversity, choice affects various axes of contextuality—gender, social, economic, geographical background, and so on—of the determinants of both child mortality and survival. Moreover, ignoring it, as we hinted, might be taken to mean a tacit acceptance of expert-driven approach to interventions, which healthcare has increasingly become, thanks to the growing preponderance of the modern allopathic healthcare system and the simultaneous decline of traditional systems of medicine. In other words, the issue of contextuality does not simply arise vis-à-vis empirical determinants of child mortality—though many are inclined to ignore that as well—but also vis-à-vis the normative determinants of child survival (that is, healthcare interventions). Even the normative should be empirically tested—what works and what does not for a particular individual or group.

However, modern healthcare tends to ignore pervasive human diversity and differential impact or side effects. Talking about the 'substantial, non-specific (heterologous) effects' that vaccines have had in high mortality areas, Sankoh et al. (2014: 645–6) argued that 'most childhood interventions (vaccines, micronutrients) in low-income countries are justified by their assumed effect on child survival'. Figure 4.6 clearly shows that vaccines are not needed to address the major causes of neonatal deaths in India—still, international donors and national policymakers have prioritized its universalization on the basis of their assumed effects. We discuss this in detail as we discuss child vaccinations among selected groups in India subsequently. For now, let us end this section by saying that, despite great strides and proliferation in access to diagnostic machines, diagnosis of the causes of illness and death tends to be superficial at best, even in the biomedical realm, not to talk of going further backwards and trying to analyse the intermediate or structural determinants of illness or death. Data sources as well as collaborative scholarship between biomedical experts and social scientists needs to be strengthened within a mutually respectable (both groups have a crucial role to play) and multidisciplinary framework.

Selected Determinants: Access or Utilization

Let us discuss the status of selected determinants of child mortality and survival for which data is available, starting with the international level.

International Level

Since its free market reforms in 1979, China has been able to lift nearly 800 million people out of poverty (defined internationally, as those living at or below USD 1.90 a day) (Sanchez 2017). It thus made a contribution of 61 per cent to global poverty decline between 1993 and 2011, thereby reducing its share of the global poor from 36 to 11 per cent during this period and leaving a mere 2 per cent of its population below poverty by 2013. India, on the other hand, could only lift 105 million of its citizens out of poverty between 1987 and 2011, actually increasing its proportion of the global poor from 21 per cent in 1987 and 23 per cent in 1993, and to 28 per cent in 2011. In 2013, China had less than 10 per cent of poor (25 million) compared to those in India in 2011 (268 million). China's spectacular performance on child survival seems hardly surprising given these figures—neither does India's, in a negative way though. Poverty situation in Nigeria actually worsened (see Table 4.1)—unsurprisingly, it only had a decline of 12 per cent in under-five deaths in the MDG period. However, Pakistan's situation is surprising—it did not do well on child mortality despite extraordinary poverty reduction. Bangladesh's poverty decline was only as good as India's, yet the former managed to perform much better on child mortality vis-à-vis the latter.

While China seems to be a classic case of socio-economic development and better health indicators, the cases of Pakistan, India, and Bangladesh—and China too—highlights the significance of political will in achieving better health outcomes. Since public health achievements are generally not made without the State playing a proactive role, whether at a few or all levels of determinants, one does not need to undertake a causality assessment to demonstrate the centrality of political will. Resources alone do not take us much far—countries like Bangladesh, Sri Lanka, Nepal as well as Cuba have achieved quite a lot in terms of health outcomes despite relatively less of them. Although public health advocates should continue to pressurize governments like India's to spend more on health—total government healthcare expenditure, that of the centre and the states/union territories (UTs) put together, has hovered around a single per cent of GDP since independence—we need to be aware of the limited role of resources and simultaneous significance of other determinants for which public advocacy is required.

Among the selected variables, youth female literacy rate—and vaccinations, as we discuss later—seem to have played a leading role in child survival in the case of Bangladesh. We know from the existing literature that maternal education contributes to child survival, and increased access to child vaccinations could be one of the pathways through which this comes to happen. China started out on a higher curve and completed its full circle with total youth female literacy. India also did very well, even though Pakistan and Nigeria did not. Youth female literacy data appears to be a strong explanation for child mortality outcomes as discussed in the last chapter.

On basic drinking water services, Bangladesh did slightly better than China, and Pakistan vis-à-vis India—with all four countries having quite high an achievement on this front. Improved sanitation seems correlated with child survival during the MDG era in the cases of China and Bangladesh, but not Pakistan though, which performed the best on this indicator, while India did only better than Nigeria. Hopefully, things

TABLE 4.1 Selected Determinants of Child Survival in Top Five Contributors to Under-Five Deaths (1990), in Percentage

Determinant	Year	India	China	Nigeria	Pakistan	Bangladesh
Poor population*	1985–90	45	67	45	59	44
	2009–13	21	2	54	6	19
Female literacy rate (% age 15–24 years)	1990–91	49	92	63	61 (2008)	38
	2010–16	82	100	58 (2008)	66	94
Use of basic drinking water services	2015	88	96	67	89	97
Improved sanitation (% of population with access)	1990	17	48	38	24	35
	2015	40	77	29	64	61
Births attended by skilled health staff	1990–94	34	94	31	19	10
	2013–14	81	100	35	52	42
Antenatal care (ANC, at least 4 visits)	2011–16	51	69	51	37	31
Postnatal care (PNC), Newborns	2011–16	24	–	14	43	32
PNC, Mothers	2011–16	62	–	40	60	36
Vaccinations: DPT3	1990	70	97	56	54	69
	2015	87	99	49	72	97

* Below international poverty line of USD 1.90 per day.
Source: WDI; ANC and PNC: UNICEF-SOWC 2017.

would improve with the 'Swachh Bharat Abhiyan' (Clean India Mission) enthusiastically launched across the nation by India's Prime Minister, Narendra Modi in 2014. Geruso and Spears (2013) have argued that better sanitation among Muslims vis-à-vis Hindus fully accounted for the child mortality differentials between the two groups at the national level. However, we also see a widespread discrimination against Muslim localities—not just backward ghettos, but also areas inhabited by educated Muslim elite, for instance, in the university town of Aligarh—in terms of cleanliness by municipalities. Garbage is not picked up for months, there are open drains, and so on. Not that this does not happen in backward Hindu and other localities too, but this is a very regular feature of Muslim localities at a more general level. Geruso and Spears instead are focusing on personal cleanliness. Let me also add with reference to the Gorakhpur deaths mentioned in the previous chapter, that several state and central ministers, all from the BJP, kept blaming lack of sanitation on parents of the dead children. Even under the Swachh Bharat Abhiyan, there has been an effort to raise awareness among and engagement of general public. That is definitely needed for the success of the Mission. However, we need to be clear that the ultimate responsibility for sanitation and cleanliness is that of the government. Citizens tend to cooperate with the proactive involvement of the government— if they are not cooperating, it is usually because they are disillusioned with the government. Despite all the hype around the Mission, there is very little that the government has actually done to raise the standards of sanitation and cleanliness in the country so far.

As far as medical interventions at primary health level are concerned, almost all births were attended by skilled health staff in China. This may have been one of the initial advantages that the country had in terms of reducing child mortality. Bangladesh and Pakistan started out from very low levels and only managed to improve decently rather than dramatically. India did best on this front, but that does not seem to be reflected well in its child survival. Nigeria did worst, which seems to be reflected in its child survival. Both India and Nigeria stood at equal levels in terms of ANC; China was the best—not highly accomplished though—and Bangladesh the worst. In terms of PNC, too, it does not seem highly correlated with child survival, although both ANC and PNC are extremely crucial for the survival and well-being of the mother and children. For newborns, PNC is particularly low in all countries, with the highest in Pakistan and the lowest in Nigeria. If we are to go beyond bare survival and be concerned about long-term well-being of children, their care at the postnatal stage in particular has to be strengthened, and so should it be at later stages—if this is the level of care at the PNC stage, it is not going to be any better at the higher levels. However, improved ANC and PNC are only possible with strong primary health systems, on which there does not seem to be much focus at a practical level, though not always in words. Finally, DPT3 vaccinations, like youth female literacy rate, discussed earlier, seem to correlate exactly with the pattern of progress on child survival among selected countries, discussed in the previous chapter. However, this correlation will be much less straightforward when we come to the selected groups in India. We, therefore, defer critical discussion to later. Nevertheless, on the whole, we again realize the contextual nature of determinants.

Inter-State Level

As one may expect, there are enormous variations in terms of the determinants of child survival and their correlations with child survival among Indian states/UTs (Table 4.2). Kerala and Tamil Nadu had the highest levels of decline in U5MR between NFHS-1 and NFHS-3—with Kerala recording the highest decline between NFHS-3 and NFHS-4 as well—and also the second highest levels of poverty decline between 1993–4 and 2011–12—with Kerala having the lowest level of poverty in 2011–12 as well as the highest level of female literacy during both NFHS-3 and NFHS-4. Himachal Pradesh recorded the highest poverty decline in the country and also had the second highest levels of female literacy during both NFHS-3 and NFHS-4—although its U5MR decline between NFHS-3 and NFHS-4 was not impressive at all, it was second only to Kerala and Tamil Nadu between NFHS-1 and NFHS-3. Household poverty decline and improvements in female literacy seem correlated with U5MR declines in most states, the former much more strongly. U5MR decline may have been higher with better improvements in the latter, an area of concern, which could also reflect limited achievements in gender (social) justice despite rapid gains in most cases at the economic level. One challenge is that it is difficult to include women aged 15–49 years (who are covered under female literacy here) in the formal education system, but that cannot be an excuse for ignoring them, especially given that their education is not only intrinsically but also instrumentally valuable. One lesson that we can draw here is that states need to do much more in terms of literacy and education of women in the childbearing age group. One quick remark before we move on—with the limited exception of Rajasthan, the other BIMARU states performed badly on both these indicators as well.

As far as other household variables are concerned, drinking water source does not seem much of a problem for most states, with the exception of Jharkhand, but it also seems to be on track with the highest improvement between NFHS-3 and NFHS-4. Despite this data, drinking water is actually a major problem in India, with no sustainable solution other than quality water purifiers, which are not easily affordable even for the middle class populations. We need to have more robust data on this issue rather than pat our backs for such assumedly high coverage. Kerala also had the highest levels of sanitation in the country, while Tamil Nadu made the highest improvement in terms of both sanitation and clean cooking fuel—there is some evidence to show their interlinkages with child survival and better health outcomes in both these states in general. However, for the overall country, major improvements are needed in terms of sanitation (except for Kerala) and use of clean cooking fuel (except for Delhi). These are two of the other major issues that are holding the country back in terms of achieving better health outcomes, particularly child survival. Central and local governments need to act much more concretely in terms of both, especially sanitation.

In terms of healthcare too, several deficits exist even in the best of states. For instance, ANC coverage in Kerala despite being the best in the country has actually gone down between NFHS-3 and NFHS-4, and continues to be quite low. In such cases, we need to be sensitive to the demands of both equity and aggregative improvements. In this case as well, we can see the neglect of gender justice and the short-sightedness of those who, almost blindly, focus on vaccinations. 'Care' is the word not just in healthcare, but more broadly—Sujatha Rao's book, *Do We Care?*—on India's healthcare is a very apt title. Nevertheless, we have done well on institutional births, with Kerala and Tamil Nadu standing at China's level, while others still have some distance to cover. But the point of institutional births, in the long term, is to develop a contact for continued care of the mother and child, which does not seem to be happening. Our primary healthcare systems are too obsessed with delivery

TABLE 4.2 Selected Determinants of Child Survival in Major States/UTs of India, in Percentage

Major states/UTs	U5MR		Household poverty as per official Tendulkar line		Literate women (aged 15–49 years)		Households with improved drinking water source		Households using improved sanitation facility	
	NFHS-3	NFHS-4	1993–94	2011–12	NFHS-3	NFHS-4	NFHS-3	NFHS-4	NFHS-3	NFHS-4
India	74	50	46	22	55	68	88	90	29	48
Bihar	84	58	61	34	37	50	96	98	15	25
Chhattisgarh	90	64	51	40	45	66	78	91	15	33
Delhi	47	47	16	10	77	82	91	86	63	74
Gujarat	61	43	38	17	64	73	89	91	44	64
Haryana	52	41	36	11	60	75	96	92	40	79
Himachal Pradesh	42	38	35	8	80	88	88	95	37	71
Jammu & Kashmir	51	38	27	11	54	69	81	89	25	53
Jharkhand	93	54	61	38	37	59	57	78	15	24
Karnataka	54	32	50	21	60	72	86	90	34	58
Kerala	16	7	32	8	93	98	69	94	91	98
Madhya Pradesh	93	65	45	32	44	59	74	85	19	34
Maharashtra	46	29	49	17	70	80	93	92	32	52
Odisha	91	49	60	33	52	67	78	89	15	29
Punjab	52	33	22	8	69	81	99	99	51	82
Rajasthan	85	51	38	15	36	57	82	86	19	45
Tamil Nadu	35	27	45	12	69	79	91	91	22	52
Uttar Pradesh	96	78	49	30	45	61	94	96	21	35
Uttarakhand	56	47	34	11	65	77	87	93	44	65
West Bengal	59	32	40	20	59	71	94	95	35	51

(Cont'd) →

Major states/UTs	Households using clean fuel for cooking		Mothers who received full ANC		Institutional births		Mothers who received PNC from a health personnel within 2 days of delivery		Full immunization (children aged 12–23 months)	
	NFHS-3	NFHS-4	NFHS-3	NFHS-4	NFHS-3	NFHS-4	NFHS-3	NFHS-4	NFHS-3	NFHS-4
India	26	44	12	21	39	79	35	62	44	62
Bihar	10	18	4	3	20	64	13	42	33	62
Chhattisgarh	13	23	6	22	14	70	21	64	49	76
Delhi	80	98	24	37	59	84	50	63	63	66
Gujarat	40	53	21	31	53	89	52	63	45	50
Haryana	30	52	12	20	36	81	39	67	65	62
Himachal Pradesh	29	37	16	37	49	76	36	70	74	70
Jammu & Kashmir	39	58	13	27	50	86	45	75	67	75
Jharkhand	11	19	5	8	18	62	16	44	34	62
Karnataka	29	55	25	33	65	94	57	66	55	63
Kerala	28	57	67	61	99	100	85	89	75	82
Madhya Pradesh	18	30	5	11	26	81	25	55	40	54
Maharashtra	44	60	15	32	65	9	57	79	59	56
Odisha	10	19	12	23	36	85	32	73	52	79
Punjab	40	66	12	31	51	91	53	87	60	89
Rajasthan	21	32	6	10	30	84	27	64	27	55
Tamil Nadu	31	73	28	45	88	99	86	74	81	70
Uttar Pradesh	17	33	3	6	21	68	12	54	23	51
Uttarakhand	36	51	13	12	33	69	28	55	60	58
West Bengal	17	28	10	22	42	75	36	61	64	84

Source: NFHS reports; Poverty: Panagariya and More (2013).

(Cont'd)

per se. We need to expand the focus of care and survival. Immunization and PNC seem to be developing fine, though, as elsewhere there are substantial disparities between states.

One interesting thing to note is the decline in PNC and immunization in Tamil Nadu between NFHS-2 and NFHS-3, despite it being the state with the highest level for both during NFHS-2. Maybe, this explains why the state did not do as well in terms of U5MR decline between NFHS-3 and NFHS-4 as it did between NFHS-1 and NFHS-3. The lesson one needs to draw from this is that even well-achieved healthcare systems need to be constantly on the vigil in terms of their existing achievements—and obviously, in terms of improving their levels. There is no room for complacency for even the best of states, especially given the weak overall environment in the country which tends to push one down rather than encourage to scale newer heights. Lastly, aggregative efficiency, or raising the overall bar, is something that we have to be perpetually concerned with. Without it, the pursuit of equity would only follow a downward rather than an upward spiral—something that we need to be cautious about in a state of extreme inequalities in particular.

Inter-Group Level

Since we are dealing with several indicators in the sphere of determinants compared to one in the case of child survival, we confine our discussion here to the national level alone without discussing the situation at the state level. However, we will refer to data from states as required.

Economic Status

Hindus and Muslims seem to be nearly uniformly represented across the wealth quintiles[26] (Figure 4.9), while nearly half of SCs and

---

[26] The NFHS-3 wealth index is based on the following 33 assets and housing characteristics: household electrification; type of windows; drinking water source; type of toilet facility; type of flooring; material of exterior walls; type of roofing; cooking fuel; house ownership; number of household members per sleeping room; ownership of a bank or post-office account; and ownership of a mattress, a pressure cooker, a chair, a cot/bed, a table, an electric fan,

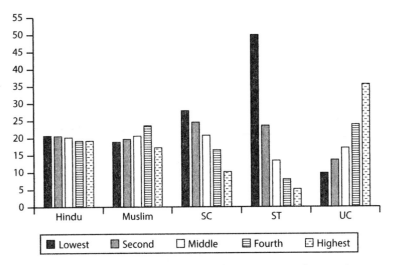

FIGURE 4.9   Wealth Index by Background Characteristics, India, NFHS-3
Source: NFHS national report.

three-fourths of STs were in the lower two quintiles, with 10 and 5 per cent representation respectively in the highest quintiles. The situation of UCs is exactly the opposite—60 per cent of them were in the upper two quintiles, and just 10 per cent in the lowest. Figure 4.10 demonstrates that a clear gradation in poverty exists between Hindus, Muslims, SCs, and STs—we do not have estimates for UCs or by gender, not for the latter since poverty in India has been measured at the household level, though there would most likely have been a strong female disadvantage if it was measured at an individual level. Not only do Hindus continuously have lower poverty, decline was also highest among them in the past two decades. On the other side, the SCs were continuously behind Muslims, but with a better decline, they narrowed the gap with the latter. STs, on the other hand, continued to perform the worst, and the gap between them and others has increased over

---

a radio/transistor, a black and white television, a colour television, a sewing machine, a mobile telephone, any other telephone, a computer, a refrigerator, a watch or clock, a bicycle, a motorcycle or scooter, an animal-drawn cart, a car, a water pump, a thresher, and a tractor.

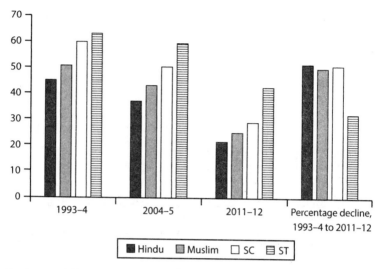

FIGURE 4.10   Poverty Among Selected Groups in India (Rural + Urban),
1993–4 to 2011–12, Based on Tendulkar Line
Source: Panagariya and More (2013).
Note: Bars on the left axis, circle on the right.

time. The advocates of free market growth in India revel over reduction in poverty since liberalization in 1991, but we need to be sensitive
to the changing patterns of inequality in this aspect—43 per cent of
STs were still poor even by national standards, which are anyways
quite low. Such inequalities in performance on poverty reduction as
well as other indicators have affected aggregate performance too. As an
aside, it needs to be noted that social, economic, and political discrimination and systemic neglect, in addition to their intrinsic importance,
are also the biggest obstacles to national growth and development
in India—something which those, always in search of opportunities to spread hatred and discord among communities, claimants of
'India First' and self-appointed defenders of national pride, should
understand. If you weaken your own people, your country will also,
eventually, be weakened. India's poor contribution to global poverty
decline is not surprising at all in the context of social prejudice, discrimination and systemic neglect—persistence of poverty in India, in
my opinion, is primarily a social rather than an economic issue, as are
most other issues that we will discuss.

Educational Status

Figure 4.11 shows clear-cut gradation in literacy rates over the past five decades by caste/tribe and by gender within each. The disparity among females has not been any better either—despite more than four times higher improvement, SC and ST females continued to remain behind their general category counterparts, started as they did from extremely low thresholds. Although ST females started out from a slightly lower level, SC females achieved the highest increase across all categories, indicating a widespread advantage among SCs in terms of benefits accruing from affirmative action policies compared to the STs. As part of their mobilization too, Dalits have championed modern education as a means of social as well as economic and political mobility. A senior Dalit intellectual and activist, Chandra Bhan Prasad, went to the extent of building up a temple for goddess 'English'! Despite better female improvement across all categories, gender inequities in literacy rates continue to be substantial, though at the aggregate caste/tribe level, there is some reduction due to better improvements among STs and SCs vis-à-vis the general category. Continuing inequities in such basic aspects as literacy rates—we are not even talking about educational attainments or quality of education—has ensured that India has

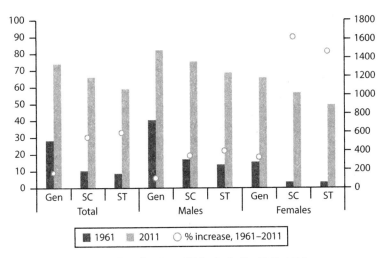

FIGURE 4.11   Literacy Rate by Caste/Tribe in India, 1961–2011
Source: Panagariya and More (2013).
Note: Bars map to the left axis, circles to the right.

struggled in such primordial concerns as child survival despite, on the other side, becoming one of the top ten economies in the world. To what extent can modern India sustainably grow without 'Bharat' (traditional India) is something we need to ponder about. Massive inequities in such basic achievements continue to hold the country from realizing its potential, not just in terms of economic growth, but also broader, and much more important, social development. Social injustice is not without repercussions for larger prosperity and growth. How STs managed to have better child survival in the 1970s, and possibly earlier, despite such low female literacy rates in particular is something that epidemiologists should ponder about. However, let us once again affirm the contextuality of determinants—in the previous section itself, we had seen how female literacy played a substantial role in child survival at the state level.

Similar to patterns which we will see in terms of utilization of healthcare, UCs were at the top and STs, SCs, and the Muslims at the bottom, worse than the national average, in terms of the educational status of women in the reproductive age-group (Figure 4.12).

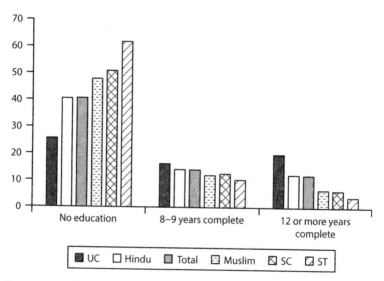

FIGURE 4.12   Percentage Distribution of Women Aged 15–49 Years by Number of Years of Education Completed, India, NFHS-3
Source: NFHS national report.

Sixty-two per cent of ST women did not have any education in NFHS-3 vis-à-vis 34 per cent ST males (Figure 4.13), highlighting gender inequality in education among STs as well, who were otherwise known for gender parity. Though the overall pattern remains similar in the case of males, SC men had an advantage over Muslim men across all categories, which shows that SC men have benefited more than SC women from affirmative action in education. Caldwell and McDonald's (1982) explanation of schooling, making parents part of the Western culture, which awards higher priority to women and children in terms of healthcare, appears plausible in the case of Muslims if we look at their access to modern healthcare, although their explanation is quite Eurocentric and debatable, given a better place for women and children in tribal communities earlier if not now. From the perspective of Muslim advantage in child survival, too, their explained pathway does not hold. The same can be said about child survival among the STs in the late 1970s and the 1980s. To avoid this Eurocentric bias in data collection, we need to have data on literacy and education in alternative systems of learning as well.

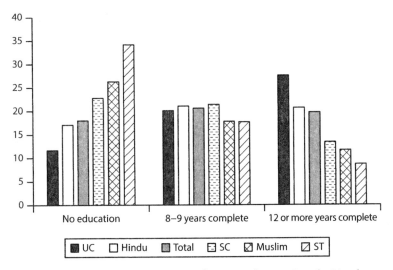

FIGURE 4.13   Percentage Distribution of Men Aged 15–49 Years by Number of Years of Education Completed, India, NFHS-3
Source: NFHS national report.

Status of Women/Mothers

Since the overall status of women/mothers at a general level as well as their health status and access to healthcare services in particular, at least a few months before and after a child's birth, are quite crucial for the health and survival of newborns, let us start with some relevant female indicators at the national level.

Women's empowerment is regarded as an intermediate determinant of child survival, and it is not difficult to appreciate its influence in the Indian context, given the general state of women's empowerment across groups (Figure 4.14). India's STs used to be characterized by much better female empowerment vis-à-vis the mainstream society, but they gradually lost their edge under the influence of the latter not

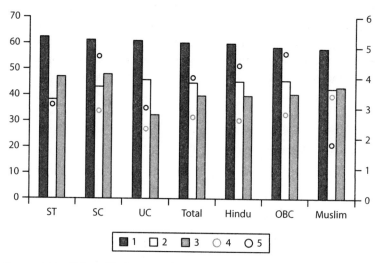

FIGURE 4.14   Selected Indicators of Women's Empowerment, India, NFHS-3
Legend:
1: Percentage of married women who usually make decisions alone or jointly with their husband for daily household purchases
2: Percentage of women who have money that they can decide how to use
3: Percentage of ever-married women age 15–49 who have experienced emotional, physical, or sexual violence by their husband
4: Total fertility rate (TFR) for three years preceding the survey
5: Percentage of women who have taken a loan from a microcredit programme
Source: NFHS national report.
Note: Bars map to the left axis, circles to the right.

only in this dimension but also child survival, as discussed in the previous chapter. Even now, although they had the highest percentage of women reporting that they usually make decisions alone/jointly with their husbands for purchase of daily household needs—followed by SCs and UCs, with Muslim women least empowered on this front—they reported the lowest percentage of women who have money which they can decide how to use, with UCs leading the group and Muslims managing to do only better than the STs. In terms of violence by husbands, SCs were slightly worse than STs, with Muslims in the third place and UC women least affected. This seems to be reflected in the total fertility rate (TFR)—that is, births per woman—on which Muslim women are the worst off, followed by STs, SCs, OBCs, and UC women once again better off than all others. On economic empowerment—percentage of women who have taken a loan from a microcredit programme—Muslim women are the worst, with UC women, surprisingly, following them, and equally surprising, OBC and SC women at the top, and ST women doing slightly better than their UC counterparts. Labour force participation rate is just 15 per cent among Muslim vis-à-vis 27 per cent among Hindu women (Census 2011).

On the whole, the status of Muslim women is worse on almost every count, which is an anomaly, like many others that we will discuss in the remaining parts of this chapter, given their much better performance on child survival. From a counterfactual perspective, Muslim children would have done much better had this not been the case. But do we not talk about the significance of female empowerment in their case when we talk about child survival? As we discuss further, both factual and counterfactual scenarios have to be taken into consideration in our discussions of justice if we are looking at optimals rather than just inter-group or individual differentials. However, let us first highlight that women, or the issue of women empowerment, cannot simply be seen from the narrow and instrumentalist perspective of reproductive and child health, which is what seems to have largely happened in India, given the focus on the specific *maternal* rather than *women's* health at a more general level. Women's health, and their empowerment, should, first and foremost, be of intrinsic concern from the perspective as well as pursuit of both justice and health. Second, given that there are only minor variations in female empowerment across social groups in India, as we just discussed, it is an issue of broader concern rather than that of a particular group alone (Muslims), which it has been made out to be—the discussion on triple talaq (divorce through three pronouncements) in the Indian Parliament and media being a case in point. It would be a folly to act like a strict egalitarian on the issue of gender empowerment in India from the perspective of groups—the issue is critical, first and foremost, from a general gender rather than a religious or a caste perspective. Having said that, the situation of Muslim women has to be taken up on top priority, and not just with respect to triple talaq, but in a much more comprehensive way—socially, educationally, economically, politically, and so on. Without their empowerment in such dimensions, we are not going to make much of a difference to their lives. However, that can rarely be expected in the given political climate in the country where the so-called concern for Muslim women is part of a wider strategy to divide and weaken the Muslims rather than to promote the empowerment and development of Muslim women.

However, true to their anomalous situation, despite being worse off than most groups in terms of empowerment, Muslim women are only behind UCs when it comes to female undernutrition (Figure 4.15). Even though STs and SCs performed the worst, Muslim women recorded the

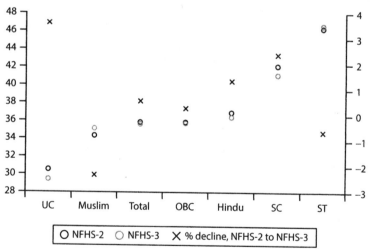

FIGURE 4.15   Among Ever-married Women Aged 15–49 Years, Percentage Who are Total Thin (BMI Less Than 18.5), India, NFHS-3
Source: NFHS national reports.
Note: Circles map to the left axis, crosses to the right. The circles for Total and OBC overlap for NFHS-2 and NFHS-3—the value in each case is 36.

worst change in their nutritional status between NFHS-2 and NFHS-3—another example of their declining comparative advantage over other groups over time, as we saw vis-à-vis child survival as well. The story looks similar when we look at anaemia among women aged 15–49 years (Figure 4.16). Surprisingly, its prevalence increased among all groups between NFHS-2 and NFHS-3, with Muslim women, once again, registering the worst change, despite only being behind UCs in NFHS-2, but falling behind OBCs by NFHS-3. ST and SC women, likewise, performed the worst. Nevertheless, if half of the women among the best-performing group (UCs) are also anaemic, it is a cause of general alarm, and we would not do justice to them or the situation of women at large if we were only worried about narrow differentials in attainment.

One can understand the limited reliance of UCs on government welfare programs like the Integrated Child Development Services (ICDS) (Figure 4.17), given that they have generally been the best group, even if in a relative sense. However, invariably lowest utilization of various categories of ICDS services among Muslims, both during pregnancy and while breastfeeding, is difficult to justify. Ordinary Muslims have, by

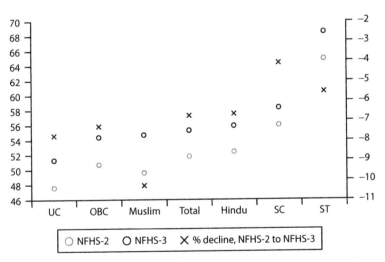

FIGURE 4.16   Among Ever-married Women Aged 15–49 Years, Percent who Have Anaemia (Less Than 12 g/dl or 11 in the Case of Pregnant Women), India, NFHS-3

Source: NFHS national report.

Note: Circles map to the left axis, crosses to the right.

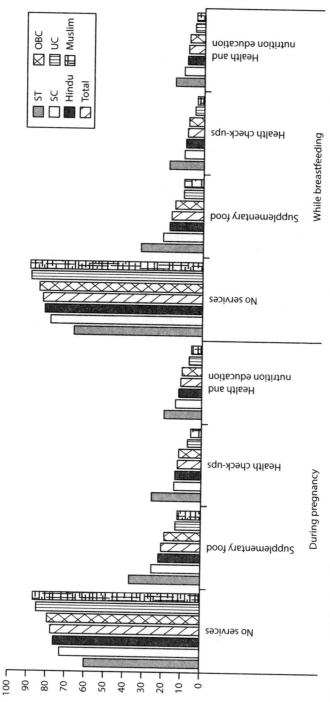

FIGURE 4.17 Utilization of ICDS Services among Mothers of Children Under Age 6 Years (%) in Areas Covered by an AWC, India, NFHS-3
Source: NFHS national report.

and large, remained alienated from the Indian state—be it political representation, positions in the public sector or welfare benefits—and this seems to be reflected very clearly in this and several other variables that will follow in this chapter. Better child survival among Muslims is not an outcome based on preferential treatment by the State—or 'appeasement', as right-wing political parties portray it to be—rather without it. Should Muslims deserve lesser treatment from the State if they are doing better on child survival? On the other hand, STs have been the biggest beneficiaries in this regard, followed by SCs—two focus groups in terms of affirmative action policies of the Indian state since independence. In their case though, worse child survival vis-à-vis Muslims is despitea preferential treatment by the State in all aspects highlighted above.

Moving on to institutional healthcare, in terms of ANC, UCs were best placed in NFHS-2 and NFHS-3 as well as improvement between these two surveys (Figure 4.18). On the other hand, although STs were worst during all three NFHS surveys, they registered the highest improvement between NFHS-1 and NFHS-2 as well as NFHS-2 and NFHS-3, and dramatically narrowed the gap with Muslims, who

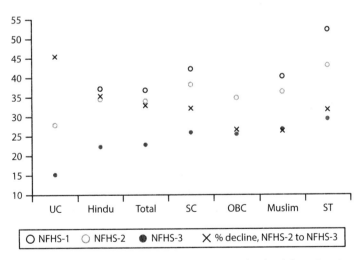

FIGURE 4.18 Percentage of Women with a Live Birth who did not Receive any Antenatal Care During Pregnancy, India, NFHS-1 to NFHS-3
Source: NFHS national reports.

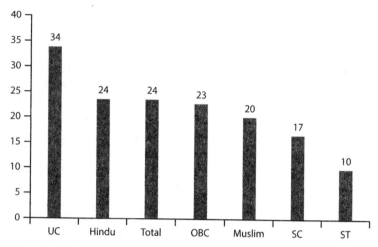

FIGURE 4.19   Percentage Pregnancies in Five Years Preceding the Survey for which Ultrasound Test was Done, India, NFHS-3
Source: NFHS national report.

registered the second lowest improvement between NFHS-1 and NFHS-2 and the lowest between NFHS-2 and NFHS-3, falling behind the SCs as well by NFHS-3. A similar pattern is visible when it comes to pregnancies for which an ultrasound was done (Figure 4.19). Prenatal ultrasounds are conducted to evaluate the progress of pregnancy as well as the health and growth of the child. However, in India, such ultrasounds are common for sex determination and subsequently abortion—their higher utilization by the more educated and wealthier sections of society is also reflected in lower sex ratio among them (see Figure 3.18 in Chapter 3). Ultrasound use among STs was lowest, and therefore perhaps not unsurprisingly, sex ratio among them was better than the average. Likewise, both the overall sex ratio and child sex ratio was better among Muslims than Hindus as per Census 2011—936 and 931 (overall sex ratio) as well as 950 and 925 (child sex ratio) respectively.

Institutional childbirths have been incentivized under RCH so that there is access to hygienic conditions as well as to trained medical staff during birth, and thereby fewer chances of delivery complications and maternal or newborn mortality. Such deliveries also help in recording births and deaths, and delivering post-birth services to mothers and newborns. Figure 4.20 shows that UCs, once again, were at the top both

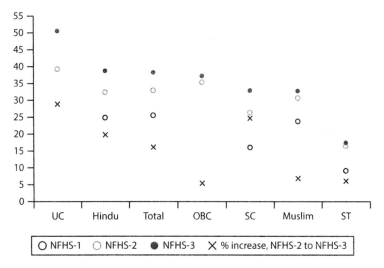

FIGURE 4.20 Percentage of Live Births in Five Years Preceding the Survey Delivered in a Health Facility, India, NFHS-1 to NFHS-3
Source: NFHS national reports.

in NHFS-2 and NHFS-3. If we look at deliveries in public and private healthcare institutions separately, they continued to remain at the top, with the highest percentage increase in both public and private sectors, particularly in latter, between NHFS-2 and NHFS-3. SCs started out second last in NHFS-1, but ended up doing slightly better than Muslims by NHFS-3, with a much higher improvement among them, second only to that of UCs. STs remained at the bottom throughout on this front, with one of the lowest increases, although slightly higher than that of the OBCs. In NHFS-3, we find exactly the same pattern as in the earlier healthcare indicators—UCs at the top, followed by Hindus, national average, OBCs, SCs, Muslims, and STs—as do we with regard to PNC in Figure 4.21. During my field visits to 10 villages in Saharanpur district of UP in 2009, I was told that there have been cases of emergency in which the concerned local public health centre refused to admit pregnant women, and they actually delivered right outside the centre. I was also told by an elderly Dalit respondent that he has seen Muslim women being humiliated at his local public health centre, which is why they preferred to stay away from their services. I have myself seen a respected private Hindu doctor in my hometown, Lucknow,

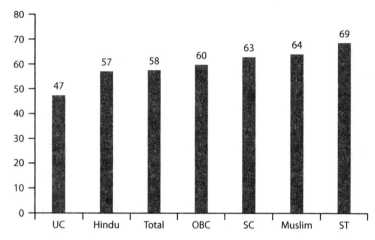

FIGURE 4.21   Percentage of Women Giving Birth in the Five Years Preceding the Survey Who Did not Receive any Postnatal Health Check-up After Their Most Recent Live Birth, India, NFHS-3
Source: NFHS national report.

UP's capital, embarrassing Muslim women—including my mother and other women I have taken there—by telling them to stop producing children! Surprisingly, despite Muslim women producing more children, they have one of the lowest percentages of institutional births in the country, which indicates the level of neglect and alienation among them—and, thanks to the rise of right-wing political parties in power, this trend is only exacerbating. Another demographic dilemma is that better child survival is supposed to reduce TFR, which again is not happening in the case of Muslims—thanks probably to lower empowerment and development indicators in general, but also, perhaps more importantly, due to religious exhortation to have more children in general, coupled with a sense of deep insecurity vis-à-vis the majority in the specific context of India.

When it comes to healthcare—or the intermediate and structural determinants of health—the situation of Muslims, as we saw, is usually comparable to that of the worst-performing groups, STs and SCs, rather than Hindus at a broader level, who almost invariably perform better than them. However, the incongruence between access to resources, on the one hand, and outcomes, on the other, does not only appear true in the case of Muslims, but STs as well—despite some of the highest improvements in terms of relevant institutional engagement, their outcomes are still the worst when it comes to child survival, while the case was just the reverse in the 1970s and possibly earlier (for which we do not have data). With better socio-economic status, UCs have been the biggest beneficiaries of RCH, substantiating Mahal et al. (2001)'s conclusion—based on their study of sixteen Indian states—that the better-off groups utilize public health subsidy disproportionately. In addition, this privilege, or the general pattern among other groups as well, is not just limited to the narrow domain of healthcare, but seems applicable to most other dimensions of structural as well as intermediate determinants of health and survival. While outcomes belied the general understanding of social inequality and gradation in the Indian context, consideration of the data on determinants supports it exactly, posing a policy and philosophical dilemma—equality of what?

Children's Status

Let us begin here with vaccinations since they have been presented as the single most important intervention not only for ensuring child survival and health, but societal prosperity in general. Basic vaccinations include one Bacillus Calmette–Guérin (BCG) injection to protect against tuberculosis, three doses each of DPT (Diphtheria, Pertussis, and Tetanus) and polio vaccines as well as one for measles. With the gender dimension now part of the data—in maternal variables, data on girl child is neither relevant nor possible to obtain—we find males as a category doing better than Hindus in general in terms of all basic vaccinations (Figure 4.22) across all NFHS surveys, even if slightly, second only to the UCs. Hindus, in their turn, did slightly better than the national average, with females worse than it. In NFHS-2, both males and OBCs stood equal, but with a positive change of 5.3 per cent in the case of the former and a negative change of the same magnitude among the latter between NFHS-2 and NFHS-3, the former took a substantial lead over the latter in NFHS-3. In the bottom rung, SCs led the group, followed by Muslims and STs in all the NFHS surveys. Despite that, between NFHS-2 and NFHS-3 in general, STs had the highest level of improvement, followed by UCs and Muslims, and then the rest. This shows that, contrary to general perception, child vaccinations have actually been picking up among Muslims, relatively more than other

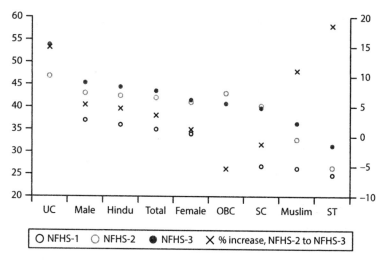

FIGURE 4.22   Percentage of Children Aged 12–23 Months Who Received All Basic Vaccinations (BCG, Measles, Three Doses Each of DPT and Polio Vaccine at Any Time Before the Survey) by Background Characteristics, NFHS-1 to NFHS-3, India

Source: NFHS national reports.

Note: Circles map to the left axis, crosses to the right.

groups. Once again, we see how one's socio-economic status (structural and intermediate determinants) plays such critical role in access to the immediate determinants, at least at the national level in India. STs and Muslims have been at the bottom of the political and economic systems, if not necessarily the social system; likewise their access and utilization of public health services has been lowest.

Nevertheless, while there seems to be some correlation between vaccination and U5MR status at two ends of the spectrum—in the case of UCs as well as the STs—its *assumed effect* is once again missing in the case of Muslims. They have the second lowest U5MR and the second lowest vaccination coverage too, although this relationship is supposed to work inversely. The impact of vaccination in other countries of South Asia is also not so clear. Figure 4.23 shows that the increase in vaccination coverage in Bangladesh was not as dramatic as the decline in IMR between 1993–4 and 2011. The same appears to be true in the context of India as well. However, Nepal, Pakistan, Maldives and Sri Lanka do show some correlation between the two. Let me clarify before we move on that

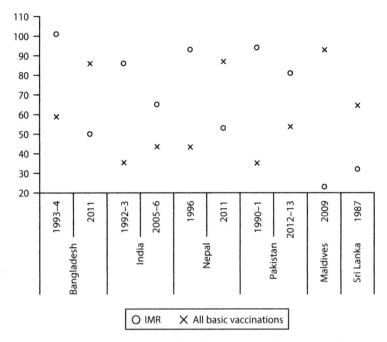

FIGURE 4.23   IMR (Ten Years Preceding the Survey) and Percentage of Children Aged 12–23 Months Who Received All Basic Vaccinations, Selected DHS Surveys in South Asia
Source: Measure DHS website.

I am not trying to prove/disprove the impact of vaccinations or other biomedical determinants of child survival, but to demonstrate that the impact of most, if not all, the determinants is contingent on variations in internal and external characteristics of individuals and groups, and therefore not uniform, or even positive in *all* cases. A deterministic approach vis-à-vis determinants is, therefore, not based on evidence and different individuals and groups might require different levels of the same intervention—and, therefore by extension, arguing for equality of access to resources in this particular case at least would not be scientific.

It is not that Muslim children need biomedical care less than others; in fact, they might actually be in more need of it given their morbidity and nutritional status, as evidenced in Figure 4.24—they had the highest prevalence of diarrhoea, acute respiratory infection (ARI), and fever, which were second highest cause of death among under-five Indian children in

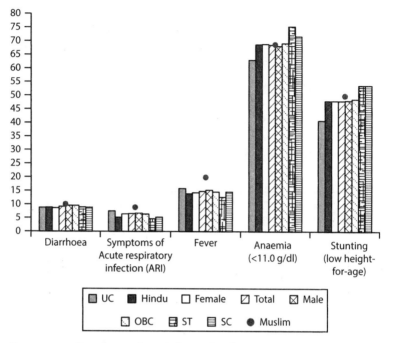

FIGURE 4.24   Prevalence of Morbidity and Malnutrition Among Children by Background Characteristics, NFHS-3, India

Source: NFHS national report.

Notes: Following are the reference groups for various categories of morbidity and malnutrition. For diarrhoea, ARI, and fever, it is the percentage of children under age 5 years in 2 weeks preceding the survey; for anaemia, percentage of children aged 6–59 months classified as having anaemia; for stunting, percentage of children under 5 years classified as malnourished as per WHO standards.

general in 2016 (IHME).[27] Surprisingly, females were the least affected in terms of diarrhoea, followed by the UCs. Males, on the other hand, were worse off than even the STs and only better than the Muslims. Once again, surprisingly, ST children performed the best on ARI and fever and UCs only better than Muslims, with females doing slightly better than males. In terms of anaemia though, we see the return of the usual trend, with UCs being the best, followed by males, national average, Hindus,

[27] Institute for Health Metrics and Evaluation, Seattle (Washington), http://vizhub.healthdata.org/gbd-compare/.

Muslims, females, OBCs, SCs, and STs. On stunting, the trend is more or less similar, with the exception that females do very marginally better than males, while Muslims, as usual, do only better than SCs and STs. Whatever the causes of their survival advantage, should Muslim children or parents, especially mothers, be discriminated in terms of access to healthcare or other determinants of survival?

The ICDS of the Government of India has aimed at the holistic development of children and pregnant/lactating mothers from disadvantaged sections particularly, by providing supplementary nutrition as well as other services through Anganwadi Centers (AWCs). AWC services for children also include growth monitoring, immunizations, health check-up, and pre-school education in addition to supplementary food. Figure 4.25 shows that Muslim children were invariably, like

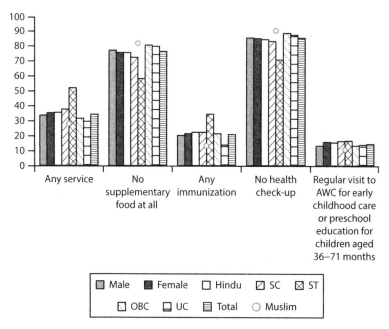

FIGURE 4.25   Percentage of Children Under Age Six Years Who Are in An Area Covered by an Anganwadi Centre (AWC) Who Received Any ICDS Service from an AWC in the 12 Months Preceding the Survey by Background Characteristics, NFHS-3, India
Source: NFHS national report.

their mothers, the lowest beneficiaries of ICDS services. As part of the Prime Minister of India's 'New 15 Point Programme for Welfare of Minorities' (NCM 2006), it was decided that a proportion of ICDS projects and AWCs should be located in blocks and villages with a substantial population of minorities to ensure that the benefits of the scheme are equitably available. SCs and STs, on the other hand, were invariably the biggest beneficiaries of ICDS services across all components. Still, they were worst in terms of nutritional status and anaemia among women and children, even as Muslims were better off than them on both. Once again, when it comes to micronutrient intake (Figure 4.26), we find the usual clubbing of groups—UCs and males on the better end of the spectrum, with STs, Muslims, and SCs on the worst end, with the exception of Muslims in the case of deworming medications, in which case their consumption was the highest.

On most of these variables, we find a pathetic performance overall, with the 'best' at best being a relative privilege, something which the

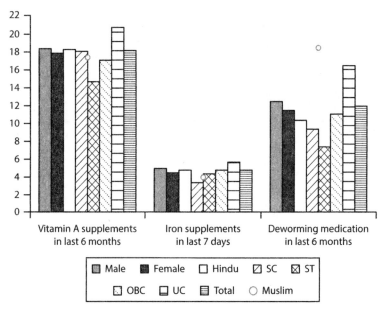

FIGURE 4.26 Micronutrient Intake: Percentage of Children Aged 6–59 Months Who Were Given the Above, NFHS-3, India
Source: NFHS national report.

best as well as the country's policymakers—many of whom come from this 'best'—should realize. Such advantage will only be illusory if we ignore the concerns of aggregative efficiency and be concerned with inter-group inequality alone vis-à-vis access or outcomes—no matter which group's perspective we look at it from. If UCs were to feel good about it, they would be mistaken; if SCs or STs were to feel that public welfare is their exclusive privilege, they would also be mistaken. Nevertheless, given the highly unequal nature of the Indian society, the pursuit of aggregative efficiency itself should be made increasingly equitable and decreasingly discriminatory. Why should certain groups only be entitled to public welfare rather than be empowered to become equal partners in the process of aggregative growth and efficiency? Historically, males and UCs have positioned themselves as the flag-bearers of aggregative growth and efficiency, while women, SCs, STs and, to some degree, Muslims have been the flag-bearers of equity. Much of the conflict in the country is in these terms. In the case of efficiency–equity trade-off, the interests of the worse off should be prioritized, as a general principle, although not always in terms of extreme priority, as Rawls would want. The pursuit of aggregative efficiency should not be made to suffer for any narrow pursuit of equity—the former should continuously raise the bar for the latter. A prime focus on differentials between the actuals and the optimals of individuals and groups, in an absolute or relative sense—that is, vis-à-vis their own specific optimal or an agreed upon threshold—should always be kept in mind as that particular approach to inequality has the potential additional advantage of improving the overall situation along with priority for the worst off in a sequential manner.

References

Arokiasamy, P. and A. Gautam. 2008. 'Neonatal Mortality in the Empowered Action Group States of India: Tends and Determinants'. *Journal of Biosocial Science* 40(2): 183–201.

Bhalotra, Sonia, Christine Valente, and Arthur van Soest. 2010. 'Religion and Childhood Death in India'. In *Handbook of Muslims in India*, edited by Rakesh Basant and Abusaleh Shariff, 123–64. New Delhi: Oxford University Press.

Bicego, G.T. and J. Ties Boerma. 1993. 'Maternal Education and Child Survival: A Comparative Study of Survey Data from 17 Countries'. *Social Science & Medicine* 36(9): 1207–27.

Black, Robert E., Saul S. Morris, and Jennifer Bryce. 2003. 'Where and Why are 10 million Children Dying Every Year?' *The Lancet* 361(9376): 2226–34.

Caldwell, J.C. 1979. 'Education as a Factor in Mortality Decline: An Examination of Nigerian Data'. *Population Studies* 33(3): 395–413.

Caldwell, John and Peter McDonald. 1982. 'Influence of Maternal Education on Infant and Child Mortality: Levels and Causes'. *Health Policy and Education* 2(3–4): 251–67.

Chattopadhyay, Aparajita, Ranjana Singh, Rajib Acharya, and Subrata Lahiri, eds. 2004. 'Influence of Non-biological Factors on Early Neonatal Mortality: Evidences from some Selected States of India'. Population Association of America, Annual Meeting Program, Boston, Massachusetts, 1–3 April.

CSDH. 2008. 'Closing the Gap in a Generation: Health Equity Through Action on the Social Determinants of Health'. Final Report of the WHO Commission on Social Determinants of Health (CSDH). Slide 2 of presentation. http://www.who.int/social_determinants/final_report/media/csdh_report_wrs_en.pdf?ua=1 (accessed 18 August 2018).

Darmstadt, G.L., Z.A. Bhutta, S. Cousens, T. Adam, N. Walker, and L. de Bernis. 2005. 'Evidence-based, Cost-effective Interventions: How Many Newborn Babies can We Save?' *The Lancet* 365(9463): 977–88.

Farmer, Paul, M. Commons, and J. Simmons. 1996. *Women, Poverty, and AIDS. Sex, Drugs, and Structural Violence.* Boston: Common Courage Press.

Geruso, Michael, and Dean Spears. 2013. 'Sanitation and Health Externalities: Resolving the Muslim Mortality Paradox'. https://www.isid.ac.in/~pu/seminar/dean.pdf (accessed 18 August 2018).

Gilligan, James. 1997. *Violence. Reflections on a National Epidemic.* New York: Vintage Books.

Government of India. 2011. Census 2011. New Delhi: Office of the Registrar General & Census Commissioner, India, Government of India.

Guralnick, L., ed. 1963. *Mortality by Occupation Level and Cause of Death among Men 20 to 64 years of Age. USA, 1950.* Washington, DC: U.S. Department of Health, Education, and Welfare.

Julia, C. and A.-J. Valleron. 2011. 'Louis-Rene Villerme (1782–1863), a Pioneer in Social Epidemiology: A Re-analysis of his Data on Comparative Mortality in Paris in the early 19th century'. *Journal of Epidemiology & Community Health* 65(8): 666–70.

Kembo, Joshua, and van Ginneken, Jeroen K. 2009. 'Determinants of Infant and Child Mortality in Zimbabwe: Results of Multivariate Hazard Analysis'. *Demographic Research* 21(13): 367–84.

Kitagawa, Evelyn M. and Philip M. Hauser. 1973. *Differential Mortality in the United States. A Study in Socioeconomic Epidemiology.* Cambridge, MA: Harvard University Press.

Krieger, Nancy. 2011. *Epidemiology and the People's Health. Theory and Context.* New York: Oxford University Press.

Kunst, Anton. 1997. 'Cross-National Comparisons of Socio-Economic Differences in Mortality'. Thesis submitted at Erasmus University, Rotterdam. https://repub.eur.nl/pub/61069/1-s2.0-S0277953698000410-main.pdf (accessed 18 August 2018).

Lawn, Joy E., Simon Cousens, and Jelka Zupan. 2005. '4 million Neonatal Deaths: When? Where? Why?' *The Lancet* 365(9462): 891–900.

Mahal, Ajay, Singh, Janmejaya, Singh, Farzana Afridi, Vikram Lamba, Anil Gumber, and V. Selvaraju. 2001. 'Who Benefits from Public Health Spending in India?'. Working Paper 56371, The World Bank, Washington, DC. http://documents.worldbank.org/curated/en/930041468285004372/pdf/563710WP0publi10Box349502B01PUBLIC1.pdf (accessed 18 August 2018).

Mosley, W. and S. Becker. 1991. 'Demographic Models for Child Survival and Implications for Health Intervention Programmes'. *Health Policy and Planning* 6(3): 218–33.

Mosley, W.H. and L.C. Chen. 1984. 'An Analytical Framework for the Study of Child Survival in Developing Countries'. *Population and Development Review* 10(Suppl.): 25–45.

Nadda, J.P. 2015. 'So Our Children May Live'. *The Times of India*, 28 April, New Delhi.

Nag, M. 1983. 'Impact of Social and Economic Development on Mortality: Comparative Study of Kerala and West Bengal'. *Economic and Political Weekly* 18(19, 20, and 21): 877–900.

Navarro, V. 1990. 'Race or Class versus Race and Class: Mortality Differentials in the United States'. *The Lancet* 336(8725): 1238–40.

———. 2000. 'Development and Quality of Life: A Critique of Amartya Sen's Development as Freedom'. *International Journal of Health Services* 30(4): 661–74.

Navarro, Vicente and Leiyu Shi. 2001. 'The Political Context of Social Inequalities and Health'. *Social Science & Medicine* 52(3): 481–91.

NCM 2006. 'Prime Minister's New 15 Point Programme for the Welfare of Minorities'. National Commission for Minorities (NCM), New Delhi. http://www.minorityaffairs.gov.in/sites/default/files/pm15points_eguide.pdf (accessed 18 August 2018).

Nelson, M.D. 1992. 'Socioeconomic Status and Childhood Mortality in North Carolina'. *American Journal of Public Health* 82(8): 1131–3.

OHCHR and WHO. 2008. *The Right to Health.* Geneva: Office of the United Nations High Commissioner for Human Rights (OHCHR) and World Health Organization (WHO).

Pega, Frank, Ichiro Kawachi, Kumanan Rasanathan, and Olle Lundberg. 2013. 'Politics, Policies and Population Health: A Commentary on Mackenbach, Hu and Looman (2013)'. *Social Science & Medicine* 93(Sept.): 176–9.

Pradhan, Jalandhar and Perianayagam Arokiasamy. 2010. 'Socio-economic Inequalities in Child Survival in India: A Decomposition Analysis'. *Health Policy* 98(2–3): 114–20.

Pritchett, Lant and Charles Kenny. 2013. *Promoting Millennium Development Ideals. The Risks of Defining Development Down.* Washington, DC: Center for Global Development (CGDEV).

Ratcliffe, John. 1977. 'Poverty, Politics, and Fertility: The Anomaly of Kerala'. *The Hastings Center Report* 7(1): 34–42.

RGI. 2009. *District Level Estimates of Child Mortality in India based on the 2001 Census Data.* New Delhi: Office of the Registrar General of India, Ministry of Home Affairs, Government of India.

Rutstein, S. and K. Johnson. 2004. *The DHS Wealth Index. DHS Comparative Reports.* Calverton, MD: ORC Macro.

Sanchez, Carolina. 2017. 'From Local to Global: China's Role in Global Poverty Reduction and the Future of Development'. The World Bank. https://goo.gl/3qMuyi (accessed 1 February 2017).

Sankoh, Osman, Paul Welaga, Cornelius Debpuur, Charles Zandoh, Stephney Gyaase, Mary Atta Poma, Martin Kavao Mutua, et al. 2014. 'The Non-specific Effects of Vaccines and Other Childhood Interventions: The Contribution of INDEPTH Health and Demographic Surveillance Systems'. *International Journal of Epidemiology* 43(3): 645–53.

Schell, Carl Otto, Marie Reilly, Hans Rosling, Stefan Peterson, and Anna Mia Ekström. 2007. 'Socioeconomic Determinants of Infant Mortality: A Worldwide Study of 152 Low-, Middle-, and High-income Countries'. *Scandinavian Journal of Public Health* 35(3): 288–97.

Sen, Amartya. 2012. *Poverty and Famines. An Essay on Entitlement and Deprivation.* New Delhi: Oxford University Press.

The Million Death Study Collaborators. 2010. 'Causes of Neonatal and Child Mortality in India: A Nationally Representative Mortality Survey'. *The Lancet* 376(9755): 1853–60.

van der Heyden, J.H.A., M.M. Schaap, A.E. Kunst, S. Esnaola I. Stirbu, R. Kalediene, P. Deboosere, et al. 2009. 'Socioeconomic Inequalities in Lung Cancer Mortality in 16 European Populations'. *Lung Cancer* 63(3): 322–30.

Wardlaw, Tessa, Danzhen You, Lucia Hug, Agbessi Amouzou, and Holly Newby. 2014. 'UNICEF Report: Enormous Progress in Child Survival but Greater Focus on Newborns Urgently Needed'. *Reproductive Health* 11(82): 1–4.

WHO. 2006. *Neonatal and Perinatal Mortality. Country, Regional and Global Estimates*. Geneva: World Health Organization.

———. 2016. *WHO Recommendations on Antenatal Care for a Positive Pregnancy Experience*. Geneva: World Health Organization.

Wilkinson, Richard G. 1989. 'Class Mortality Differentials, Income Distribution and Trends in Poverty 1921–1981'. *Journal of Social Policy* 18(3): 307–35.

5

Which Shot of Justice?

M ost of us are aware of the divisions and discriminations that have characterized Indian society at a broader level. It was, however, quite astonishing for even me to see them reflected so vividly in most of the indicators that we discussed in the previous two chapters, especially those concerned with access to resources. Two things are very clear from this data. One, child mortality is primarily a problem of social injustice, both from an equity and an efficiency perspective. Social injustice is not only responsible for inter-group inequities, which have come out so clearly in the data that we have discussed here, but also for keeping aggregative achievement low, particularly vis-à-vis the positive potential that the country and its citizens possess.

Economically, the country is now among the top ten economies in the world; socially, it continues to be among the worst. As the old English proverb goes, 'united we stand, divided we fall'. If our energies are concentrated on multiple axes of divisions and discriminations, we are not only weakening others, but also undermining the wider social contract and, as a result, the potential of collective achievement and bargaining that enables citizens to pursue their collective rights in a democracy. The politics and practice of social injustice has only aggra-vated the situation by favouring certain groups and excluding others based on such grounds which are neither fair nor rational, be it from a political philosophical, policy, or public perspective. Two, because of its structural underpinnings, child mortality is not just a biomedical issue that can be tackled solely through shots of vaccinations or other such biomedical interventions. Even within that narrow realm, access and utilization have very clearly been patterned based on social injustice. Children as well as their parents need a shot of justice not just to survive, but realize their optimal potentials. The question remains—which shot of justice is best suited for this purpose? Grounded in the empirical context of the Indian society, let us now invoke major theories of justice to respond to this question.

Equity in Relevant Indian Policies

Since one of our objectives has been to inform the design and assessment of child survival policies from an equity perspective, let us start out by analysing the understanding and approach to equity of relevant Indian policies in the context of child mortality. While there has been no specific policy of child survival, five policies of the Government of India have dealt with the issue in some measure—the National Policy for Children (NPC) of 1974 and 2013, and National Health Policy (NHP) of 1983, 2002, and 2017.[1] As we discover, all of them have largely focused on equality of opportunity/resources, predominantly with reference to healthcare and early nutrition, even if they have referred to the structural determinants of child survival. One could argue that a typical health policy can, in fact, only go so far. Structural and intermediate determinants of child survival in particular, health and well-being in general, have to be addressed through multisectoral action, with the ministries of finance playing a central role through adequate resource

[1] Two ministries in the Government of India have been largely responsible for the health and survival of children—the Ministry of Women and Child Development (MoWCD), which is the nodal ministry for coordinating the implementation of the Convention on the Rights of the Child 1989 and for the formulation and monitoring of NPCs; and the Ministry of Health and Family Welfare (MoHFW), which is the nodal ministry for most health-related issues and provisions as well as for the formulation and monitoring of NHPs. Earlier, the Ministry of Human Resource Development played a leading role—it not only brought out the NPC 1974 as well as the National Charter for Children in 2003 (NCC 2003), it also established the Department of Women and Child Development in 1985. This department was later upgraded into the MoWCD in 2006. Given the interlinkages of maternal and child health and development, it made sense to have an independent Ministry devoted to them together.

allocation. However, one could also argue that no matter how multi-sectoral the action is, the ministries of health—and by extension health policies—have to coordinate public action on health with the engagement of not just a whole range of public agencies and ministries, but various actors concerned with, or with an impact on, children's/citizens' health.[2] The ultimate responsibility for health outcomes should rest with the ministries of health—obviously, with adequate powers to fulfil this responsibility. However, the NPCs—focused as they were on children, with a whole-of-government and whole-of-society approach—could have dealt with structural and intermediate determinants of child survival and well-being and the mechanisms through which they could have been addressed. To be fair to them, nonetheless, both NPC 1974 and 2013 did take a holistic view of child development in contrast to the MoHFW, which has remained focused only on child survival within an immediate biomedical framework, that too narrowly on vaccinations. It makes sense that children's overall growth and development remain the primary responsibility of the MoWCD, but this should be accompanied by a clear and consistent focus on child survival and well-being, which does not seem to be the case at the moment. However, let us move forward to assess the framework through which the relevant policies have approached the issue of equity in the context of child survival. As mentioned earlier, these policies are not exclusively child survival policies and have also been concerned with other issues; however, given our focus here, we confine ourselves to their equity aspects vis-à-vis child survival. Let us begin with NPCs since they have been more directly concerned with children's welfare.

---

[2] In reality, however, we have seen that tobacco and food industries, for instance, hold considerable clout in policy circles, and are able to have people in the MoHFW, at times even ministers of health themselves, removed if the latter act in a manner that is prejudicial to their vested interests. Policymaking in the real world is about balancing a host of competing interests, and health usually has one of the weakest constituencies, especially in rapidly developing countries like India, where economic growth and GDP figures almost assume a divine and non-negotiable status. This only demonstrates the powerful influence of the structural determinants of health and of child survival, of the centrality of political will, otherwise how could countries with a lower GDP per capita than India—China of a few decades back and Bangladesh even now—could have achieved in terms of child survival what India has not been able to so far.

NPC 1974

Recognizing children as 'a supremely important asset' of the nation, the NPC 1974 identified 'their nurture and solicitude' as 'our responsibility'— it is not clear whether 'our' refers to the Government of India or the country as a whole. Such lack of clarity on responsibility of children has been a characteristic feature of Indian policy, though various government documents have paid lip service to the significance of children as a national asset. One could expect such clarity at least from a national policy dedicated to children. Nevertheless, this policy was extraordinary from at least two perspectives.

One, in qualitative terms, the NPC 1974 went beyond bare survival (in terms of outcomes) and immediate determinants (in terms of resources)—that, too, at a time when child mortality was way much higher than it is now and the pressure to tackle it much higher. It argued that 'all children in the country enjoy optimum conditions for their balanced growth', for 'full physical, mental and social development', and acknowledged that 'rise in the standards of living, wherever it occurred, has indirectly met children's basic needs to some extent'. Given that it was formulated in socialist India, there was commitment to children's holistic growth as well as recognition of challenges related to wider development and social justice in this regard. Post-liberalization, the focus in terms of outcomes and recognition of determinants seems to have largely been reduced to the immediate. Another case of policies being socially determined, by the dominant ideology and political orientation, at both the national and international levels. As a final comment, let me state that, in terms of action, the NPC 1974's focus seems largely confined to healthcare and nutrition only, although it did talk about multisectoral action and coordination—another example of Indian policies being high on promise, and low on commitment and action.

Two, the NPC 1974 considered 'all' children deserving of 'equal opportunities for development'. For shortfalls within a general 'equality of opportunity', it talked about 'special assistance' to 'the weaker sections of the society', which, from its perspective, included children of SC, ST, and economically weaker backgrounds in urban and rural areas. The socialist government of that period saw this well-aligned with its 'larger purpose' of 'reducing inequality' and bringing about 'social justice'. This approach also appears to make a lot of sense from the perspective of Rawlsian/resourcist theories of justice, though the latter were by no means socialist in their orientation. Why such an approach to justice is inadequate—even if not irrelevant—is discussed in the next section, but let us look at the selected target groups here.

Let me begin by saying that including *all* children under its purview of equality of opportunity was a revolutionary step since even children of otherwise privileged background can be disadvantaged in certain respects, as we have seen in the data presented in the previous two chapters. Justice for children has to be *primarily* concerned with children themselves, not parents or their backgrounds. In this sense, justice for children has to be justice in the most inclusive of forms, especially because we cannot assign responsibility for particular actions or outcomes to small children who are under consideration here. Nor can they be held responsible for the background or actions of their parents. To do so would be utterly unjust. But so was it to include *all* SC and ST children, despite regarding economically weak background as the third criterion for special assistance—which itself is, at best, a proxy for children's health, but not a definite measure or one of intrinsic value as far as children's well-being is concerned. What about children requiring 'special assistance' from other groups, or those from these two groups not standing in need of it? Indian policies have rarely been able to go beyond the framework of historical, caste-based or 'social' injustice, doing enormous injustice to non-targeted groups and individuals within them. Justice has been pursued on political rather than principled or political philosophical grounds.

Secondly, injustice and discrimination in India are not just based on caste/tribe or economic status—what about inequity and discrimination based on religion, for instance, directed against Muslims? Inequities based on religion have rarely been on the Indian policy radar, with the time around the Sachar Committee Report (2006)[3] being one of the notable exceptions. The report of the Post-Sachar Evaluation

---

[3] It was a high-level committee constituted by the then Prime Minister of India, Manmohan Singh, with a mandate to study the social, economic, and educational status of India's Muslim community. Its very formation and a subsequent statement by him at the 52nd meeting of the National Development Council that minorities, especially Muslims, 'must have the first claim on resources' (8 December 2006, New Delhi) led to a major backlash and counter-mobilization.

Committee—which was constituted by the previous government at the Centre to take stock of changes since the release of the former report, and for which I wrote the health chapter—was rejected by the new government on the pretext of its overarching slogan, '*sabka saath, sabka vikaas*' ('together with everyone, for everyone's development'). Even citizenship rights of Muslims are perpetually questioned, not to talk of their claims to justice. In January 2018, an eight-year-old Muslim girl was gang raped over several days until she died, and the bar council in that part of the country was not even allowing an advocate to take up her defence, instead coming out openly in support of the accused, who happened to belong to the majority community. The first challenge for Muslims is to be acknowledged as victims of social injustice—which is further complicated given their widespread perception as 'terrorists', and anti-Muslim hatred being a global norm—which is not a concern as far as SCs, STs, women, or the economically weak are concerned.

The criticism of exclusion of Muslims from the purview of special assistance is largely a general one rather than directed at NPC 1974 alone. Despite their focus on equality of opportunities, even if in the limited space of healthcare, Muslims have been ignored in all policies under consideration, though there are some measures in place for the education of Muslim girls, economic empowerment, and so on, in minority-oriented policies. The public narrative and policies on social justice in India have led to exclusionary and competitive tendencies—beneficiaries want to exclude as many as possible, while excluded assertive communities have been demanding, at times violently, to be included in the list of 'backward' communities entitled to reservations in government jobs and other domains. The aggregative failure of the government in job creation has taken a turn towards counter-claims of social justice. In China, massive poverty declines following the free market reforms happened because the government was able to engender rapid urbanization and structural transformation of jobs from agriculture to industry, which has largely eluded India so far. Even here, the approach of the Indian government is to shirk its responsibility.

In the midst of all these sociopolitical churnings and more than 70 years after India's independence, Muslims are still struggling to be recognized as rightful citizens of the country. Efforts have been made to keep Muslims on the back foot through issues of cross-border terrorism and infiltration, international terrorism, and so on, and to portray them as aggressors, who should be ashamed of themselves rather than be claimants of victimhood or justice. Nay, they should accept all injustices against them without complaining. Like survival and health, policies have social determinants of their own. We have tried to illustrate the context in which not just NPC 1974 in particular, but various policies have excluded Muslims from claims to justice.

NPC 2013

Coming after a gap of almost 40 years, the NPC 2013 adopted a rights-based approach and argued that 'the right to life, survival, health and nutrition is an inalienable right of every child and will receive the highest priority'. Unlike NPC 1974, it focused on *negative discrimination*, in a libertarian sort of tone, by proclaiming that 'no child shall be discriminated against on grounds of religion, race, caste, sex, place of birth, class, language, and disability, social, economic or any other status'. Like NPC 1974, it argued for 'equal opportunities' and a comprehensive approach to child development—the 'mental, emotional, cognitive, social and cultural development of the child is to be addressed in totality'. Although it took note of potential challenges at the level of intermediate determinants and took a radical stand—'no custom, tradition, cultural or religious practice is allowed to violate or restrict or prevent children from enjoying their rights', 'special measures and affirmative action are required to diminish or eliminate conditions that cause discrimination'—like NPC 1974, when it came to action, it fell short of expectations, settling for the immediate 'equitable access' to healthcare and a 'right to adequate nutrition'. Even these belittled promises have largely remained hollow—the previous two chapters provide evidence on the same. The focus clearly has to be on, as Amartya Sen argued, 'actual injustices', especially in a context like India, lest policies make us delusional about the grand promises of justice.

Nevertheless, one significant aspect of NPC 2013, which is closer to the capability approach, is its recognition that 'every child is unique', and that 'children are not a homogenous group and their different needs need different responses, especially the multi-dimensional vulnerabilities experienced by children in different circumstances'. However, this does not seem to reconcile well with its 'equal opportunities' approach since different children would require different/unequal opportunities in different contexts for their 'multi-dimensional vulnerabilities' to be addressed. It reconciles even less so with its advocacy of equality in terms of access to healthcare—if vulnerabilities are multi-dimensional, should not the pursuit of equality as well be multi-dimensional/multi-sectoral? There is recognition of the need for multisectoral action in most policies, but when it comes to equity, they tend to timidly confine themselves to the narrow space of healthcare and nutrition. Likewise, how does the right to life reconcile with its equal opportunities or the more limited equal access to healthcare approach? Ensuring every child's right to life or health, given that every child is unique, as the policy itself acknowledged, could mean very unequal opportunities or access to healthcare, and by advocating the latter, the policy is actually undermining its central promise, the right to life.

NHP 1983

It is impressive to find a health policy starting out with reference to the constitutional ideal of the 'establishment of a new social order based on equality, freedom, justice and the dignity of the individual'. While equality, freedom, and justice were part of the official narrative of the socialist regime of that time, reference to the *individual* is significant, given the focus on *social* (caste) and class-based justice. While it went on to recognize that 'poverty and ignorance are among the major contributory causes of the high incidence of disease and mortality', the beginning was also the end of engagement with the notion of equality. All one can make of in terms of equity was 'cent percent coverage of targeted population groups with vaccines'[4]— limited even within the already narrower space of healthcare, despite all its lofty references—'a special focus on the less privileged sections

---

[4] This is despite its criticism of 'Western models, which are inappropriate and irrelevant to the real needs of our people and the socio-economic conditions obtaining in the country' and praise for India's 'ancient medical systems' as 'holistic' (NHP 1983). Or maybe the authors of this policy believed that vaccines were invented in ancient India, as is the predominant belief among Hindutva forces regarding several modern inventions. In that case, one can only wish that we had realized the significance of vaccines earlier and saved millions of children.

of the society', and first priority in services 'to those residing in the tribal, hill and backward areas'. The latter aspect of the policy seems to have been successful to some degree—healthcare coverage among tribals has definitely gone up.

Nevertheless, though the Emergency imposed by the Central government from 1975 to 1977 was officially over by the time this policy came out, obsession with population stabilization was clearly not. Despite recognizing that 'a vicious relationship exists between high birth rates and high infant mortality', it accorded 'the highest priority' to maternal and child health as a result of this 'vicious relationship'. And rather than calling for a separate National Child Survival Policy—that may have helped in the reduction of child deaths, and thereby of high rates of fertility and population growth—it instead called for a separate National Population Policy, which too came only 17 years later, in the year 2000. Policymakers in India seem to have been concerned with the sociopolitical ideals of equality and justice, but also seem to have struggled in terms of conceptualization as well as operationalization of these ideals. Policy advisers have not done any better either, concerned as they have been almost exclusively with the technocratic rather than visionary aspects of policymaking.

NHP 2002

The NHP 1983 started out on a promising note, and the NHP 2002 ended with one. It referred to equity as 'one nagging imperative' which had influenced every aspect of it, an 'independent goal' based on which its success or failure was to be judged in the future rather than on an aggregate or financial measure. However, like other policies, its concern for equity was restricted to 'more equitable access to the health facilities'. In line with our findings in the previous chapter, it felt that 'access to, and benefits from, the public health system have been very uneven between the better-endowed and the more vulnerable sections of society', and accorded 'overriding importance' to 'ensuring a more equitable access to health services across the social and geographical expanse of the country'. Though acknowledging 'inter-sectoral contributions to health', it argued that 'inter-connected sectors ... while crucial, fall outside the domain of the health sector', and that 'sectoral policy documents' like itself must 'serve as a guide to action for institutions and individual participants operating in that sector'. It did not even mention the term 'coordination', with inter-connected sectors, with health sector at the helm.

Further, within health services, it argued that primary health was the level at which 'inter-regional' (rural–urban, inter-state) inequities and those 'between economic classes' can most cost-effectively be addressed, and likewise argued for higher public health allocations for it, for the extension and improvement of primary health infrastructure and services. While it referred to inequities based on gender and caste, it did not explicitly regard Muslims among 'disadvantaged sections of society'.

NHP 2017

Equity is one of the ten key policy principles of NHP 2017, but what is unique is its acknowledgement that a 'high degree of inequity in health outcomes and access to healthcare services exists in India', with a focus on 'attainment of the highest possible level of health and well-being for all at all ages'. Indian policies have usually promised equitable access on some narrow dimension of healthcare, so a focus on outcomes, with a comprehensive view of health in terms of scope within a life course perspective, is very welcome. In another place, it talks of achieving 'optimum levels of child and adolescent health', reminiscent of Aristotle's 'human flourishing' and Sen's 'capability approach'.

Another unique feature of NHP 2017, unlike NHP 2002 in particular, is its bold acknowledgement of wider determinants of health, both in terms of their influence and the need to act on them, through evaluation of 'the impact of existing and future non-health sector programmes and policies through the health lens', institutionalized intersectoral coordination and action at national and sub-national levels in the spirit of emerging 'Health in All' approach,[5] and a 'Swasth Nagrik Abhiyan—a social movement for health'. Such an acknowledgment in the context of child survival has been even rare—'maternal and child survival is a mirror that reflects the entire spectrum of social development', and, as such,

---

[5] 'This policy recognizes the causal links between health outcomes and social determinants of health. ... Achievement of national health goals would require addressing all the social determinants (distal and proximal) ...'.

it 'aspires to elicit developmental action of all sectors' for maternal and child survival.

In terms of target groups, it talks about identification of 'the deprived areas/vulnerable population groups (including special groups) through disaggregated data' as 'a first step to address the existing inequities in health outcomes between and within States in India'. This is based on its realization that 'even in States where overall averages are improving, marginalized communities and poorer economic quintiles of the population, especially in remote and tribal areas, continue to fare poorly'. Therefore, 'demarcating areas/populations with low coverage, is a precursor to identification and removal of barriers in the underserved areas/population'. In principle, this is not only a welcome step towards evidence-based policymaking on equity, but also leaves room for the inclusion of all and not just pre-selected groups in the pursuit of justice and equity in the broader space of health.

However, despite all its uniqueness, the NHP 2017, like its predecessors, seems to fall into the trap of limited healthcare in terms of vaccination when it comes to mention of specific equity action—'for instance, fully immunized children aged 12–23 months in Odisha were only 45% in scheduled tribes as compared to 62% for the State'—and the neglect of even limited healthcare disadvantage based on religion—'reducing inequity would mean affirmative action to reach the poorest. It would mean minimizing disparity on account of gender, poverty, caste, disability, other forms of social exclusion and geographical barriers.' Muslims would, once again, miss the health equity bus despite one of the lowest utilization rates even from the perspective of the limited domain of healthcare. If Muslims were not acknowledged in terms of health inequities until now, one could not expect so from a health policy legislated under a right-wing government at the Centre. State health policies are supposed to be developed within the overall framework of the Union health policy—despite health primarily being a state subject—and so what better can one expect from them?

It is clear that, despite showing promise, child and health policies in India have ended up in timidity as far as their conceptualization and operationalization of equity and justice are concerned. Health inequities, in fact, have never been taken seriously, even at the inter-state level, despite such inequities being an explicit concern of centralized policymaking in India at a more general level until very recently.

How do we analyse these policies and develop some lessons for an equitable one in the background of discussions that we have had on theories of justice as well as the data on outcomes and access? The following discussion also has wider relevance for the pursuit of equity and justice in the space of health and more broadly for discussions of justice in political philosophy, particularly on the issue of equalisandum, as we try to illustrate in the subsequent sections of this chapter.

What Needs to Be Equalized?

Given the centrality of the question, 'equality of what?', in discussions of justice and equity, let us begin with an assessment of various proposals on the preferred metric of justice from the specific perspective of child survival. What do we owe our children—equality of opportunity, of outcomes, of capability, or equality vis-à-vis a multifocal variable which combines these seemingly disparate but independently important concerns? Because the first position is the most prominent, let us start out with it. We can make a further distinction here between equality of opportunity vis-à-vis access to immediate determinants of child survival or healthcare, as the above policies have largely done, and equality vis-à-vis the social determinants of health, including but not restricted to healthcare. Let us begin with the equality of healthcare approach.

Equality of Healthcare

One could make a number of arguments both in favour as well as against equality of opportunity in terms of healthcare. On a positive note, since healthcare belongs to the realm of immediate determinants, it is relatively easy to trace the origins of poor health outcomes to it and address it in the form of cost-effective interventions that are also measurable and immediate in terms of their impact—without affecting the status quo. Given the empirical and normative ease that the space of equality of healthcare offers, it is not surprising that most government policies as well as approaches to health equity and justice tend to concentrate on it. Policymakers and donors trying to demonstrate a quick impact with fewer resources find it particularly helpful. Because of these attributes, their case becomes even more compelling in countries like India where the target population is massive and resources—I would prefer to call it *political will* because where there is a will, there are resources—limited. However, their conceptual and interventional ease does not make the task of equality in this space any easier.

On a critical note, three major arguments can be raised. One, access or the utilization of healthcare, especially in countries like India with a high degree of systemic inefficiency and inequity, depend in several cases on, for instance, the local power dynamics (structural determinants) or parental education (intermediate determinants), even if we were to leave out the negative role of poor household wealth status which equality of opportunity in healthcare is supposed to neutralize. A higher utilization of healthcare by UCs vis-à-vis all others makes sense in this background.[6] In one way or another, we would have to deal

---

[6] During my 2009 fieldwork in UP, I asked members of various castes about access to doctors and health services of a particular health facility in their village. It was one facility, but answers varied dramatically by caste, demonstrating how there can be no single assessment of the performance of health or other facilities in the country without reference to the background of its intended users. The village facility, by the way, was locked and looked deserted when I visited it. Since it happened to be a Jat-dominated village, a group of Jat youth told me with pride that doctors at the health facility are so good that they visit 'our' houses when a member of the family falls sick and even send medicines at home. A group of Dalits, on the other hand, who were accompanying me, mentioned that, as I could see for myself, the healthcare facility was closed and even when it was open, doctors misbehave with 'us', which is why they rather preferred to go to private doctors in towns, where they were at least 'treated with respect'. Humiliation and self-respect (*swabhiman*) have been central themes in Dalit mobilization, particularly in UP, and they are relevant in the space of health as well. This is also a clear illustration of the local power dynamics playing a role in the access/utilization of health services, which is not really surprising since most doctors are from the upper castes in states like UP and are well-connected with the local dominant caste elites. In a democratic country, numbers do not always matter in the establishment of a dominant caste—in one village, there were only four Rajput families and an overwhelming majority of Dalits, yet as the local priest told me, nothing happens in that village without the approval of these families. Although its seat was reserved for Dalit candidates in local elections, one who enjoyed the patronage and 'blessings' of these families could get elected—the majority of the voters were agricultural labourers in the farms of these families. Health systems do not

with intermediate and structural determinants. Two, even if we were to deal with systemic inefficiencies and inequities, and ensure equal access to a particular system of healthcare—the predominant one being modern biomedical healthcare, to which most advocates of equality of healthcare subscribe and most governments and donors push for—it would be parochial and paternalistic to ensure equality in access to it at the expense of alternative systems of healthcare, which at least some individuals may wish to utilize rather than, or in addition to, modern healthcare. The denial of choice vis-à-vis the non-Western healthcare systems would be especially untenable given the evidence on advantage in child survival among STs during the 1970s and Muslims more or less generally, with least access to modern healthcare, which could also be construed as an argument in relative support of their own systems of healthcare. Three, as discussed in the chapter on determinants, human diversity, and differential needs based on such internal and external diversity makes the assumed effect of at least certain components of Western—for that matter, any—healthcare nonspecific so that an equal dose of healthcare may not work for all equally. Data in the previous chapter shows that assumed effects of PNC, ANC, institutional deliveries, and vaccinations are muted or missing in the case of Muslims particularly. van de Poel and Speybroeck (2009) have shown differences in the *effects* of determinants in the case of SCs and STs as well.

India's leading cardiologist, Dr Naresh Trehan, had this to say in one of his columns: 'As a disease does not behave the same way in different individuals, the response to treatment and outcome will also be variable and, therefore, it happens that with the same disease some people recover and some don't.'[7] Human diversity makes conversion of any input into expected outcomes complex. However, such a criticism is not meant to negate the utility or contribution of modern, or any other system of, healthcare—just that, none of them can be equalized in

---

work in a clinical vacuum—we need to understand their local contexts and accordingly develop policies and measures aimed at reducing inequities in the space of health. Even the narrow space of healthcare is riddled with social inequity—there are really no short cuts to flourishing, unless you lower the bar to bare survival, which, too, is not always easy.

[7] Naresh Trehan. 'When trust is at issue between doctors and patients, healing takes a backseat'. *India Today*, 20 October 2014, p. 60.

terms of access or utilization, given their differential requirements and impacts, and therefore accepted as a metric of equity and justice based on which health and survival policies could be designed or assessed.

In discussions of justice, an understanding of the scientific is also important at one level, and healthcare of any type should be judged on the basis of its efficiency—efficacy of interventions in varying contexts and cases—and not on the basis or purpose of equity and justice. To expand options (for efficiency) and choices (for equity), there is strong case for epidemiological and medical pluralism here, which NHP 2017 in particular did focus on—not least due to the desire of the RSS to revive ancient Indian/Hindu culture, Ayurveda and Yoga being its elements. Governments should make provisions for systems of healthcare customized in the light of local epidemiology and people's preferences while making them aware of their respective benefits and shortcomings so as to enable informed choices. Nevertheless, it would be out of place to demand equality in the space of any system of healthcare, not least because a chosen space should be permanent rather than one based on shifting scientific understanding. For instance, earlier, Vitamin A supplementation was shown to have a benign impact on child survival, and it was likewise incorporated in the maternal and child healthcare basket of several countries. Later, based on several experiments in Asia and Africa, its effect proved to be doubtful and two of its earlier proponents themselves argued that 'we must now focus on alternative strategies to improve the nutritional status of populations at risk of deficiency in vitamin A and other micronutrients' (Haider and Bhutta 2014). A chosen metric of justice should be sensitive to scientific understanding, but cannot exclusively rely on it.

Given human diversity, even within a family, while external characteristics of various members would more or less be the same, their internal characteristics would most likely differ and one specific package of healthcare may not work for all of them. Of course, there will always be a common set which would more or less work for most people, if not all. The Finnish government has been providing a baby box with 48 items to all expecting parents since 1938 'to start a life with a baby'.[8] We can treat that as Rawls' 'social primary goods', which every rational person might need, irrespective of whatever else

---

[8] https://www.finnishbabybox.com/en/ (accessed 28 August 2018).

he might need to attain his objectives. However, that Finnish box or Rawlsian set of social primary goods would, in fact, be quite primary, and beyond that, the package would have to be customized as per individual need and choice. No matter how much we might idolize it, primary healthcare too would not be sufficient by itself. We would have to move beyond.

Equality of Resources (General and Specific)

Major approaches under consideration here would be that of Rawls in political philosophy, Marmot's, and that of social epidemiologists' generally. The biggest problem with the approach of both Rawls and Marmot is that unless systemic changes are carried out, demands of justice would not be met from their perspective. For example, Rawls, in his book *A Theory of Justice* (1971: 7), argues that, 'for us the primary subject of justice is the basic structure of society, or more exactly, the way in which the major social institutions distribute fundamental rights and duties and determine the division of advantages from social cooperation. By major institutions I understand the political constitution and the principal economic and social arrangements.' To be fair to him, Rawls developed his approach for justice at a general and broader level and not for justice in the limited context of child survival, one may argue. However, systematic and persistent patterns of child mortality are one of the symptoms of social injustice—Rawls' ultimate prescription may therefore not be very different. Marmot also talked in a broader breath as Rawls (CSDH 2008). Thousands of children under the age of five die each day, and we cannot wait for structural determinants to be taken care of before we start saving these children, though such an approach may sound thorough and convincing from the perspective of addressing the root causes of inequity and injustice, and should actually be taken seriously from this perspective. However, as far as child mortality is concerned, such an approach is the other extreme of the healthcare approach, which focuses entirely on immediate determinants.

If the subject of justice of this approach lies in the sphere of structural determinants, its metric of justice relates more to intermediate determinants, which like immediate determinants, could play differential roles in various contexts, although, again, their role in child survival is critical. If there are substantial variations in the influence of antenatal and delivery care by country (see Figure 4.5 in the previous chapter), there are also variations by education and wealth status (Figures 4.2 and 4.3 in the previous chapter). In fact, mothers with secondary or higher education in Zimbabwe recorded a higher IMR than those with no education, and there was no differential at all in terms of IMR between those in the highest and the lowest wealth quintiles in Swaziland, and limited in the case of Zimbabwe and Moldova. We saw in the previous chapter how poverty declines among selected groups between 1993–4 and 2004–5 were largely commensurate with their U5MR declines, demonstrating a positive correlation between the two. But such a relationship did not hold in terms of education as far as Muslims were concerned—they were doing worse than national average and Hindus in terms of education, but better in terms of child survival. If some individuals and groups are able to do better with fewer resources, how do we justify the equality of resources, especially so when there might be others who might need more resources to achieve the same set of outcomes, particularly those which are of primary interest to us (like child survival in our case, in comparison to secondary outcomes like education and wealth)?

A focus on resources, intermediate or immediate, gives a resourcist and redistributive orientation to justice, though softer issues like inefficiency, corruption, discrimination, respect, and so on, which are not always dependent on resources, but more on political, economic or social arrangements, are equally, or at times more, important as far as justice is concerned. Systemic inefficiencies and corruption, for instance, affect the poor more than the rich; that should be a cause of concern as far as discussions of justice are concerned. Part of the capability-deprivation of Dalits, and also probably their shortfall in child survival, has arguably resulted from denial of self-respect and self-confidence to them by the dominant castes over centuries. Kanshi Ram, the founder of BSP as well as of large-scale Dalit mobilization in UP and, to some degree, Punjab, used to argue that 'poverty and deprivation among Dalits is the result of social and political powerlessness historically rooted in the Brahmanical system and not an economic condition to be dealt with by economic policies' (Pai 2004: 1143). According to World Bank's *Moving out of Poverty* study, even after controlling 'for a wide range of factors, the individual's own self-confidence, sense of power, and aspirations for the future emerge as a significant factor influencing mobility' (Kapoor et al. 2009: 211). It is, therefore, appreciable that, in the Rawlsian system of justice, 'self-respect and a sure confidence in the sense of one's own worth is perhaps the most important primary good' (Rawls 1971: 396). However, such a focus is missing from other resourcist approaches to justice, and Sen too has not accorded it its due. Sen also sounds resourcist in some senses when he emphasizes 'conversion'—for him, it is not about equality as such, but differential access to *resources* according to individual requirements and potentials. Nevertheless, his approach seems much more appropriate with a focus on issues of central and ultimate significance—achievements, capabilities, and human flourishing—in the context of pervasive human diversity.

Furthermore, equality of opportunity is proposed as a metric of justice largely because individuals have choice and responsibility, which is the intermediary variable that reflects on outcomes in addition to—and constrained by—the availability of resources at our disposal. However, in the case of child survival, under-five children can neither exercise choice nor be held responsible for their outcomes. To an extent, their parents can be. Nevertheless, responsibility for child survival eventually passes on to the State under two circumstances in particular. One, in a negative context, when the State takes upon itself the responsibility to prevent and even punish parents for actions that are considered harmful for survival of children (for example, female foeticide). Two, in a positive context, it is obliged to provide support to parents who are not able to take care of their children. The latter responsibility of the State should not be restricted to the financial incapability of parents, but should also include *educational incapability*, for instance—illiterate parents, even if rich, lack in health awareness and may not be able to take care of their children appropriately, thus high child mortality rates even among the rich in BIMARU states where overall literacy levels are low. In countries like India, where it becomes difficult to even hold the parents responsible, either due to their poverty or illiteracy, and if the State is supposed to play the leading role, equality of resources in the context of child survival does not mean much. Why not just equalize child survival itself, which is also of central rather than derivative significance as resources, in such situations in particular? Particularly so because State support to parents would have to be differential based on their status, and therefore the central concern would be with child survival de facto, even if not explicitly acknowledged.

Equality of Outcomes

It is much easier to have a universal consensus on survival than on its determinants, given that the former has intrinsic vis-à-vis the instrumental value of the latter. Although the right to life meant right to the 'means of subsistence and security' for Rawls, he had argued that human rights like the right to life 'cannot be rejected as peculiarly liberal or special to the Western tradition', or as 'politically parochial' (Rawls 2008: 65). As Rawls argued, the intrinsic value of survival is, further, universal compared to the contextual nature of determinants that we discussed in the last chapter. So, equality in the space of outcomes (child survival) would appear to be a natural choice as far as considerations of equity or efficiency are concerned.

However, even equality of outcomes cannot be an appropriate metric of justice due to reasons of epidemiology, equity and efficiency. From the perspective of the former, despite our best efforts, we may *unfortunately* not be able to save each and every child—for reasons beyond our capacity or control, the prospects of preventability, which would be contextual, as they fall in the space of determinants. Deaths which are not preventable would not be inequitable either—the literature on equity and justice too has made a difference between justifiable and unjustifiable inequalities, the former referred to as *inequalities* and the latter as *inequities*. Even in the Rawlsian framework, as part of his second principle of justice, inequality of opportunities should be arranged such that they 'enhance the opportunities of those with the lesser opportunity'. However, if we were to retain or promote the respective optimal capabilities of individuals or groups, equality of outcomes would mean depriving those with biological (females) or possibly cultural (STs, Muslims) advantages, as in our case, in child survival. 'Equity in survival between females and males does not imply equal mortality rates ... where boys and girls have the same access to resources ... boys have higher mortality rates than girls during childhood' (UNPD 2011: xv). Bhalotra, Valente, and van Soest (2010: 123–4), on the basis of their multivariate analysis, show how 'Muslim-status is associated with a 1.6 percentage point reduction in neonatal mortality', even after controlling for a 'rich set of covariates' as well as 'mother and village level unobserved heterogeneity'. A focus on outcomes fixates us on actual rather than potential achievements, and from that perspective, not only makes equity and justice a negative, unimaginative and uninspiring concern, but casts poorly on aggregative concerns too, which in the Rawlsian framework does not have priority over equity.

Nevertheless, one could argue for equality in outcomes as per optimals of preventability as well as optimals of groups or individuals vis-a-vis child survival, given its intrinsic importance. Different individuals/groups would need different levels of resources to achieve this equality, which is fine. However, we would still have to ask—would it be fair to provide less resources to those with a natural advantage in survival, especially with the counterfactual view that they could do better with equal resources—no group has achieved perfect outcomes as of now? This brings us to the need for a multifocal variable and focus on the individual within groups—survival of each child, irrespective of background, should be assigned equal value. However, let us not forget the competing concern of aggregative efficiency and achievement, on which again, equality of outcomes, unifocal in its approach like equality of opportunity, is lacking. We shall refer to this position as we discuss further.

A Multifocal Variable?

Although it sounds intuitive that Sen's approach would call for equality of capabilities, he does not.[9] In fact, he does not favour 'absolute priority' to any 'unifocal criterion', and argues instead in favour of equity considerations being broad, inclusive, and multidimensional. He talked of females' 'biological potentials, given symmetric care' (Sen 1995), and, therefore, from his perspective, health equity has to be sensitive not just to

---

[9] 'The capability perspective does point to the central relevance of the inequality of capabilities in the assessment of social disparities, but it does not, on its own, propose any specific formula for policy decisions. For example, contrary to an often-articulated interpretation, the use of the capability approach for evaluation does not demand that we sign up to social policies aimed entirely at equating everyone's capabilities, no matter what the other consequences of such policies might be' (Sen 2009: 232).

outcomes, but also to capabilities, *with equal access*. Therefore, it 'includes concerns about achievement of health and the capability to achieve good health, not just the distribution of health care. But it also includes the fairness of processes and thus must attach importance to non-discrimination in the delivery of health care' (Sen 2002). Sen not only takes us away from deterministic fundamentalism—for him, the *use-value* of determinants arises from their contribution to child survival, and therefore our central focal variable should be primarily sensitive to the latter rather than to the former—but also from any insistence on a single variable for all contexts and purposes. Although Sen has argued for a central place for capabilities in assessments of equity and justice, let us discuss the issue of the applicability of the chosen metric as well as preferred measurement of justice for a clearer understanding of Sen's complex position.

The Applicability of the Central Focal Variable

Since this is a 'case-implication critique' (Sen 1979), based on data for selected groups in India, for the purpose of choosing a central focal variable that is appropriate for an equitable and efficient policy of child survival, there are a number of contextual specificities in the analyses presented here, and one may raise a number of questions. For example, would the central focal variable we choose here be specific to the Indian context—or more specifically to selected cases of selected groups in India—and not be universally applicable? Would it be specific to considerations of child survival, and not be applicable to other considerations of survival or health (for example, maternal survival or health), not to talk of non-health considerations (for instance, an education policy)? Individual responsibility of outcomes, central to considerations of justice, does not apply to children under the age of five years, but would be a key variable when we discuss the survival and health of their mothers, for instance. However, there are overlaps when we discuss elementary education, for example, since we would again be talking of children to whom individual responsibility may not necessarily apply. Nevertheless, the specificity of survival in our case study would still remain, though the concerned population group would overlap in this case. There could be other specifities beyond country, sector, population group, and so on. The important question is—do they make the relevance of the central focal variable chosen here contextual rather than universal?

If yes, then even the question, 'equality of what?', which Sen argued is a central question that we need to address in considerations of equality, would itself not cut much ice,[10] unless we append such specifities to this question. For instance, should we rather be asking—*equality of what, for child survival, in India?* Sen seems to have partially addressed the issue from the perspective of purpose-, if not country-, specificity. He argued that 'inequality is measured for some *purpose*, and the choice of space as well as the selection of particular inequality measures in that space would have to be made in the light of that purpose' (Sen 1995). In the context of basic capabilities like survival, he had also argued that functionings—on which data is more readily and reliably available—could well be a good guide to underlying capabilities. However, specificities like country or age group, as far as I am aware, have not been discussed either by Sen or others, in the context of their implications for the selection of a central focal variable, although Sen did talk of looking at procedural fairness as well, in addition to health capabilities and achievements, invoking biological female advantage in survival and certain forms of illnesses.

> Within this broad field of health equity, it is, of course, possible to propose particular criteria that put more focus on some concerns and less on others. I am not trying to propose here some unique and pre-eminent formula that would be exactly right and superior to all the other formulae that may be proposed (though it would have been, I suppose, rather magnificent to be able to ordain one canonical answer to this complex inquiry). My object, rather, has been to identify some disparately relevant considerations for health equity, and to argue against any arbitrary narrowing of the domain of that immensely rich concept. Health equity is a broad discipline, and this basic recognition has to precede the qualified acceptance of some narrow criterion or other for specific—and contingently functional—purposes. The special formulae have their uses, but the general and inclusive framework is not dispensable for that reason. We need both. (Sen 2002)

Since here we are concerned with health, we can confine ourselves to his approach to health equity, without worrying that he may not

---

[10] 'In fact, equality, as an abstract idea, does not have much cutting power, and the real work begins with the specification of what is it that is to be equalized' (Sen 2002: 660).

have raised similar concerns in the context of general discussions on justice and equality, or in discussion of other sector-specific concerns, and has generally over-emphasized the space of capability over other equity considerations, especially vis-à-vis access to resources. He has also made his position on the determinants of health clear, and the broad sweep of changes that health equity may imply beyond a narrow focus on healthcare. What is particularly relevant for the purpose of our current discussion is his emphasis on non-exclusivity and case-specific considerations of health equity. Elsewhere too (Sen 1995), he says: 'The argument for paying greater attention to functionings (or capabilities) in assessing inequalities of well-being (or of freedom) must not be seen as an *all-purpose* preference for those variables.' We do not have to insist or worry about having to choose one focal variable which is equally applicable in all contexts—our selection could be context-specific.

Having said that, I would like to point out to the fact that Sen himself has adequately emphasized Aristotle's notion of 'human flourishing' as the most primary concern and goal of political activity, and this notion could well serve as *the* overarching variable, irrespective of contextual specificities. No matter what country, sector, age group, gender, and so on, we are dealing with, we could always ask at a broad level—is this particular policy, social arrangement, and so on, promoting or obstructing human flourishing (or that of concerned age group and gender, for instance)? The response to this question would inevitably be broad-based, taking into account various facets of human flourishing. For our particular consideration, for instance, it would mean looking at the overall flourishing of children, rather than the narrow space of bare survival at the neonatal or even at under-five age level. Simply bringing children to the brink of survival would not be adequate from this perspective. Even within the narrow confines of health—even if we do not talk about their education, for instance—we will have to look at their overall health, growth and development, potential of their future progress, and so on. Survival and health are the most critical aspects of human flourishing, without which it would not mean much, and therefore health has a special significance and rightly deserves a government- and society-wide 'health in all'[11] approach to take care of it.

---

[11] http://www.who.int/healthpromotion/frameworkforcountryaction/en/ (accessed 28 August 2018).

One final, broad comment before we move on. Sen's focus on pervasive human diversity and the conversion of resources into capabilities, and eventually functionings, could perhaps have been inspired by the particular Indian context—which would not be surprising given his background—where pervasive diversity is the norm, and so are institutional inefficiency and non-institutional obstacles, in varying degrees, which limit the scope of individual responsibility. On the other hand, Rawls's focus on procedural fairness could have been inspired by his own Western context, where problems specific to the Indian context are not, at least, as major an issue, and procedural fairness on its own could take us a long way in the realization of capabilities that Sen is concerned with, providing space for exercise, and accountability, of individual responsibility. If we keep perfecting the rules of the game and keep making them fairer, we might ensure that there are little systematic inequities between and within groups. Obviously, there are profound institutional as well as non-institutional challenges in developed countries too, as the experience and the situation of African Americans, for instance, demonstrates. Is the Rawlsian approach workable in the Indian context? Not in the foreseeable future, it seems. So we should basically focus on capabilities or even outcomes, given the insidious ways in which institutional and non-institutional inefficiencies and discriminations act. This might seem to be a plausible contextual explanation for the focus on different metrics. Nevertheless, we also have to acknowledge the fact that human diversity, and the resultant problem of conversion (from resources to capabilities/achievements), is not simply a matter of context—although their intensity probably is—but a universal phenomenon, and there would be internal variations (gender, age group, genetic propensities, and so on) as well as external variations which would make the relevance of these metrics universal rather than simply parochial.

Preferred Measurement of Justice

In line with his insistence on taking cognizance of pervasive human diversity and the objective of human flourishing in the pursuit of justice, Sen argues in favour of the respective *maximal potentials* of individuals as the prime comparator for the measurement of *shortfall inequality*—our respective inequalities in shortfall or distance between our actual achievements and our respective optimals. However, for him, this does not mean that we should completely ignore *attainment inequality*—inequalities vis-à-vis each other's actual achievements (between individuals/groups, for instance) or the distance between our actual achievements and a common threshold. In both cases, one could argue for applying Rawls' *lexicographic maximin*—assign priority to the interests of the worst off and try to make them as well off as possible. An exclusive focus on attainment inequality leads us to ignore pervasive human diversity and the respective flourishing potentials of individuals, groups and countries, for instance, and consequentially undermine aggregative flourishing in the name of (simple) equality (levelling-down effect), which should not be the case as equity cannot be our sole concern (Sen 1995), or—contrary to Rawls's standpoint—a priority concern over efficiency in all cases. Aggregative and efficiency concerns also have implications for the pursuit of equity—they raise the comparator even for the pursuit of attainment equality, not to talk of improvements in the general conditions of living. Second, neither the pursuit of justice nor public policy in general can ignore those who are better off, given their potentials to do better.

A focus on maximal potentials makes the agenda of equality look more positive than the traditional focus on inequalities in actual achievements between groups defined by various axes (class, caste, region, religion, and so on), which seems to qualify the definition of equality as jealousy. Most literature on health inequalities falls in this category. We could address inter-group inequalities in a positive way by trying to reduce the gap between respective maximal optimals as much as possible through supplementary focus on those whose maximal potentials are lower. In other words, there would be a double focus on the worse off in terms of the: (*a*) gap between their actual achievement and their maximal potential; and (*b*) the gap between their maximal potential and that of the better off. Both gaps should be addressed. For instance, Figures 3.34 to 3.40 from Chapter 3 of this book tell us about intra-group differentials at the inter-state level, while Figure 3.41 compares their lowest U5MRs, their best possible achievement, within the country. If we were to adopt the latter as their maximal potential within the country in the given circumstances—though we would have to explore other options that could be considered as maximals—we can focus on both issues as given in (a) and (b). Since SCs and STs have the worst lowest common denominators in Figure 3.41 (squarely due to historical injustices that they have faced), the differentials in given lowest common denominators of SCs and STs in particular vis-à-vis others are unjust and there is a strong case to further reduce the gap between their lowest denominators vis-à-vis that of others. Such an approach could ensure redressal of persistent inequalities without sacrificing the potential of better-off groups as well as aggregative concerns. It is interesting to note that females also have the lowest common denominator of all groups—which should be the case ideally—given their natural advantage in survival over males. Another interesting aspect is equal lowest common U5MRs among Hindus and Muslims, and, most importantly, the fact that most lowest denominators are from Kerala—a state which has consistently done better than other states in aggregative terms. A focus on raising aggregative achievement, as we said, raises the bar of equity comparators too.

An equitable child survival policy does not mean that we should be concerned with the *survival of the unfittest* only, though concern with them should be the highest. Systemic inefficiencies affect the better off as well. Figure 4.3 shows that IMR is by no means ignorable even among the richest. In Nepal, for instance, despite remarkable overall improvements, IMR was substantial among those in the highest wealth quintile (that is, 40). Likewise, Figure 3.38 shows that U5MR is high among the UCs too—going up to 109 in Bihar, which is worse than those in lowest wealth quintiles in Zimbabwe, Nepal, Haiti, India at the national level, Congo, Pakistan, Uganda, and Cambodia around the same time-period (Figure 4.3). Just because these children are dying among relatively privileged groups does not mean we should ignore them, even though we would give more attention to the worse off. Every child has a right to life, irrespective of background, unprivileged or privileged. If 'the aim should be to bring the health of those worse off up to the level of the best' (CSDH 2008: 29), what about progress of the best, unless we are talking about the pinnacle of achievement at the universal or absolute level? Concern with the status and performance of the better off, even if limited, should be a part of our equity considerations as they too can be held back from their respective potentials.

From this perspective, the setting up of a common proportional reduction target for all countries, irrespective of their background, under the MDGs (with MDG 4 focusing on two-thirds reduction in child mortality) was a reasonable step as all of them were expected to improve in an equal proportional sense, implying an absolute higher reduction among the worse off vis-à-vis the better off, which in turn means that inequalities between them would reduce over time. Figure 5.1 illustrates that by way of example: three countries with extremely unequal starting points (in 1990) achieve an equal percentage decline (of 68 per cent) by 2013; the higher the starting point, the higher the level of absolute reduction, which, in turn, leads to substantial reductions in attainment inequality between these three countries. While this approach looks very convincing in a situation where international consensus needs to be developed with clear operational targets, it does not pay attention to differential optimal capacities of nations, though it does not stop them from growing further and does look into cases where growth has been lower than the expected target.

Nevertheless, like any fixed measure of progress, it is not concerned per se with those who have already achieved the target or the kind of inequalities that persist within and between those above the threshold. One corrective measure to take care of this internal distributional

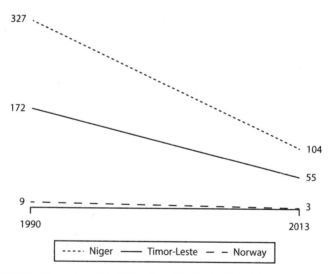

FIGURE 5.1   Countries with 68 Per Cent Decline in U5MR Between 1990 and 2013
Source: IGME.

problem would be to make this sort of target (not necessarily the particular MDG 4 target) applicable not just to countries at the aggregate level—as was the case, and the criticism of the equity-insensitive nature of the MDGs—but to all subnational units (state, districts, and so on) as well as groups (by gender, class, caste, religion, and so on) within each country. Such an approach may help in reducing inter-group inequalities, for instance, with a focus on those whose maximal potentials are lower, but will not be particularly sensitive to those whose optimals are higher (for example, female natural advantage in survival or a cultural advantage among STs and Muslims vis-à-vis others).

Critics have argued that fixed thresholds are defined in arbitrary and ambiguous ways and there is no plausible answer to 'how much is good enough?', or what should happen beyond the threshold, 'the indifference objection' (Arneson 2006). Ruger (2009: 88–91) suggests the use of an 'optimal average' or 'maximal average achievement'— for example, world's highest life expectancy—as a comparator for the measurement of respective shortfalls and achievements in different countries, and advocates a hybrid of sufficientarianism (bringing all up to a particular threshold, determined by society) and prioritarianism (a greater priority to the relative gains and losses of the less advantaged), with shortfall inequality as 'the primary methodology and standard of equality'. Although this approach appears less complicated than Sen's—determining maximal potentials of individuals will be quite complicated, while the maximal average achievement is a given which can be readily available as a target for sufficientarian purposes)—it does not seem concerned with the progress of those at the top, who would have further potential to improve, although Ruger is concerned with the respective maximal potentials of individuals and groups. However, unless we apply the *fair innings* argument (Williams 1997) to those at the top—that they have already reached a level beyond which it is not necessary for us to care about them—we may find it difficult to justify such an approach. However, a threshold beyond which no further progress is possible might seem to be a convincing proposal.

As far as the specific case of child mortality is concerned, my own suggestion is to set 'zero' as the ultimate aspirational comparator for all, calculate the respective shortfalls of countries, states, groups, and so on, from zero—with priority-setting and resource allocation commensurate with the level of shortfall. Such a comparator would neither be liable to the charge of being arbitrary since we should be making our best efforts to not let even a single child die anywhere in the world. As part of those efforts, we should probe why children are dying wherever they are, and whichever deaths are preventable, we should take it as our immediate moral duty to prevent them. If they are not preventable, we should muster resources and develop mechanisms, technologies, whatever it takes to save as many as we can. This is what most parents would do—do anything to save their children—and if they are not able to, it is the ultimate responsibility of the State to do so. If they are having more children than they or the State can afford to nurture, that is also generally the fault of the State—lack of socioeconomic development being responsible for both high mortality and fertility rates—hence the responsibility of the State to extend the frontiers of prevention with all capabilities it can optimally muster. Starting from the premise of available resources is inadequate on at least three counts: One, resources are not always the most critical determinant of child survival. Two, resources are fungible and we could leverage more resources from other sectors to save the lives of children (it is difficult to imagine anything else that could be more important—the primacy of child survival is justified on several counts). Three, when they are committed to, governments do make all efforts to mobilize resources internally and externally, and there is no reason why they should not do it to save children (most donors or countries would be happy to give at least a loan, if not grant, for the purpose of saving children). If despite our best efforts, we cannot save a child, it could be attributed to the muted maximal potential of that child within the framework of our current capabilities, while we continuously make efforts to enhance our efficiency and capability level to save each and every child. Such an approach, while ensuring the maximal survival of all, as a dynamic pursuit through extending the frontiers of prevention, would avoid the controversy of determining varying optimal potentials as well as dealing with inequalities above the threshold—the 'good enough' would be zero child mortality, nothing less. Rather than specifying a rate of reduction for international goals like the MDGs earlier and SDGs now, international agencies should start setting zero targets (with zero tolerance) for child mortality, poverty and similar ills that continue to plague human existence despite unprecedented growth and inequity reductions. They need to demonstrate the will to do so.

In the context of child mortality, another question to be asked is: reduction of what—rate or number of child deaths? Rate is a standardized number which is helpful for inter- and intra-country/group comparisons, calculated on the basis of per 1,000 live births, and the population sizes of concerned countries and groups, therefore, do not matter for the purpose of comparison. India's rank in terms of the rate of under-five mortality was 53 in 2016 (UNICEF 2017)—which does not seem too bad to us, given that there are 52 countries doing worse, including Pakistan (20)—but in terms of number of such deaths, India has held the top slot since 1953, the first year since data on under-five mortality for India is available. In accidents or calamities, we report absolute number of deaths, which makes them sound horrific. Why should not we do the same in the case of child deaths, given that they are unjust and morally reprehensible, which accidents or calamities are not, in the strict sense of the terms? From an aggregative perspective though, a World Bank (2004: 7) report on MDGs in India did argue that from a 'welfare (and policy) perspective, it may be important to attain the largest reduction possible in the absolute number of infant deaths in the country'. We can argue the same from an equity perspective too—every preventable child death is unjust, even if the U5MR in that country or group is just 1. However, when it comes to priority-setting and resource allocation, if number of deaths is the sole criterion, minority populations may get a raw deal unless there are disproportionately more children dying among them vis-à-vis the majority population, among whom number of deaths is also likely to be higher in a country doing poorly in an aggregate sense. If it actually comes to it that they deserve equal or higher priority vis-à-vis the majority with reference to the number of deaths, it would actually mean a disastrous situation among the former because that would be highly disproportionate given their population size.

Minorities are mostly vulnerable to discrimination at various levels, and such an approach would have the potential to exacerbate rather than address any relevant discrimination. This is one of the issues in the context of which it would be possible to convincingly argue in favour of an individual-rather than a group-centric approach to child survival. Priority-setting and resource allocation should be done in a way that we assign equal value to the survival of each and every child, irrespective of background. One possible approach from an aggregative perspective could be that we prioritize the focus based on the number of deaths, while from the perspective of justice, we prioritize the focus based on rate since that could potentially also keep in view the respective maximal potentials of various groups.

Most importantly, from the perspective of justice as the dynamic pursuit of human flourishing, we owe much more than basic survival to our children. The massive multidimensional inequalities that children continue to be born into—without being in any way responsible for them—is the biggest blot and challenge for the theories and pursuit of justice and equality. Yet children continue to be ignored in discussions and policies of justice and equality. Beyond vaccinations and other such basic interventions, we owe justice and fairness to every single child in this world—that is the spirit that should inspire international goals on children. In such advanced nations as the US and Israel, more than 20 per cent of children continue to live in poverty (OECD Family Database). Children even in relatively well-off countries and groups need a shot of justice. National and international agencies and policymakers should stop 'defining development down' (Pritchett and Kenny 2013), and continually raise the bar of equity and justice for one of the most vulnerable sections of the society, the future of our society—settling for nothing less than human flourishing. This is what we owe our children. This is what justice in the case of children means.

What does justice specifically mean for children from selected groups whose cases we discussed in the previous two chapters? Before we go on to discuss the wider implications of our discussions here for political-philosophical discussions and public policy on justice, let us quickly consider the case of some of these groups, and how Indian policymakers concerned with children should ensure justice for them. However, let me reiterate that justice, in the final assessment, would be individual, with several interventions at the aggregate group level to enhance the capabilities of the group as a whole as well as aggregative achievements. Aggregative considerations have to go hand in hand with equity concerns at multiple levels, from international to national, state as well as group levels. There are things that the international community, as a whole, can do to ameliorate the condition of the worst off groups and individuals around the world, for instance. The conceptualization and operationalization of justice is to be multidisciplinary and multisectoral as well as multilateral and multinational to some degree, even if most of the action has to happen at local levels. Fair trade is one idea which has the potential to ameliorate the situation of a wide variety of communities and individuals in several parts of the world. There are implications of international actions for local pursuits of justice. Action cannot just be individual, even if assessment in the final analysis should be. Despite his strong focus on the individual—'each person possesses an inviolability founded on justice that even the welfare of society as a whole cannot override' (Rawls 1971: 3). Rawls wanted to develop 'a theory of justice that generalizes and carries to a higher level of abstraction the traditional conception of the *social* contract', one in which justice was 'the first virtue of *social* institutions', 'the basic structure of society' was 'the primary subject of justice' (1971: 7) and which was focused on a fair distribution of the '*social* primary goods' (1971: 62) (emphasis added for all instances). Rawls (2008: 81) even argued for 'forceful sanctions and even 'intervention' by the international community against outlaw states that violate human rights, which does happen, although not for the right reasons in most cases, given the politics of power that insinuates such sanctions or interventions. Nevertheless, as action within a country is straightforward and uncontroversial, let us discuss what policymakers in India owe to children of some of the selected groups as far as their flourishing is concerned.

Females are said to have a biological advantage in survival, which was visible in India too during the late 1950s (Figure 3.11), and is still at the neonatal level (Figure 3.14). However, as data shows, female children lose their survival advantage, over time and over the life course, as the two figures respectively demonstrate. However, they continue to have it even in sub-Saharan African countries (Figure 3.13), and even if we ignore data from developed nations which also points in this direction, we can still adopt female survival advantage as a norm which needs to be accepted and promoted. Attainment equality with male children— worse so, inequality at this basic level—is, therefore, an instance of historical injustice to female children and policymakers need to undertake affirmative action to correct such historical injustice as they have done for SCs and STs more generally—in a similar spirit, though not necessarily in terms of content.

In terms of sex ratio, too, the same holds—policymakers are alarmed at sex ratios lower than a 100; even 100 is unjust, given their survival advantage, as a result of which the natural sex ratio at birth should be around 105.[12] Here as well, females lost their advantage over time in India (Figure 3.16). Although the national sex ratio always remained below 100 since Census 1901, four states had sex ratios over 105 in 1901, including the BIMARU state of Bihar (106)—this number went up to five between 1921 and 1941; but, in 2001 and 2011, it was just Kerala (106 and 108). The more the tribals came into contact with the mainstream Indian society, the more they got affected with its attitudes towards females and, inter alia, its sex ratio—they had above optimal average sex ratios in the early decades of the twentieth century, but lost their advantage over time. Hindus and Muslims in Kerala in 2001 had above optimal average sex ratios, which again, highlights the importance of aggregate achievements with an equity focus.

Several policy conclusions can be drawn here. One, female survival advantage needs to be restored both from a historical and a life course perspective. Two, though women have a universal biological advantage in survival, there could also be an additional cultural advantage, which tribal women in India, for instance, appear to have possessed. While a broad consensus on restoration of biological female advantage seems plausible, the restoration of the additional cultural advantage is somewhat complicated to argue for, but cannot be allowed to go waste, either from an equity or an aggregative efficiency perspective. If some individuals or groups are capable of achieving more for themselves and relevant aggregates—and one could also include the so-called upper castes here—should their optimal potentials be left unrealized, particularly with human flourishing being the ultimate goal? For sure, we should break up the ultimate goal into smaller goals—for instance, child survival until the age of five, at neonatal level, and so on. However, by the same logic, there also has to be a movement from these smaller goals towards the ultimate goal, which does not seem to happen. In other words, there are arguments to reduce the focus to neonatal mortality, as we saw in the third chapter, but we rarely hear about increasing the attention span of child survival policy from under-five to the quality of survival until this age as well as survival, health and flourishing at higher age groups—the official definition of 'child' being anyone under fourteen years in India and under eighteen years as per the UN Convention

---

[12] http://www.searo.who.int/entity/health_situation_trends/data/chi/sex-ratio/en/ (accessed 30 January 2018).

on the Rights of the Child (CRC), to which India is a signatory. And one cannot argue that we will deal with one level (neonatal or under-five) completely and only then move on to higher levels—there can be simultaneous, differential approaches for various groups, as there is already toward geographies, with an eye on raising overall achievement, and the overall bar for equity, which has to be dynamic.

While the reduction of inter-state disparities has remained a central policy principle of the Government of India since Independence, it did not mean that the higher development potential of certain states was ignored—it was, in fact, encouraged through numerous incentives and allocations. While zero child mortality, as discussed earlier, could be the negative goal of public policy in the case of child survival on the one side—according to one account, *zero* was invented in India, so let policymakers use the new-found zeal for ancient Indian inventions and leverage it in the context of child survival—there has to be a positive goal as well. It could well be the extension of the age groups of focus in terms of survival, health and flourishing, at least for those in whose case it is possible, to begin with. And when this happens, we would also have more to catch up on the equity front, for those who would not be there yet. This is probably too dynamic and unsettling for the thoroughly status quo*ist*, quintessential Indian policymaker—but so be it. We need to flag issues from a conceptual perspective, and when more and more people discuss it, it might one day enter the policy narrative too. Here I am reminded of an Urdu couplet by Muhammad Iqbal, the greatest poet-philosopher of the Indian sub-continent during the late nineteenth and early twentieth century—'*Khud badalte nahin, Quran ko badal dete hain; huwe kis darja faqeehan-e-Haram be-toufeeq*' ('They do not change themselves, rather change the Quran; how incapable have the jurists of Mecca become'). Not religiously though, the principles of justice should guide policymaking rather than the realities of policymaking setting the bar for discussions of justice.

This second issue, of cultural/community advantage, also relates to the child mortality status of STs in general as well as that of Muslims who managed to do better than others for a long time despite some of the worst access to various levels of determinants. From an aggregative as well as an equity perspective, it is also relevant for the so-called upper castes, whose situation has, in most cases, been the best both in terms of access and outcomes—but they still perform poorly overall despite the potential to perform better. Several individuals from these castes also perform poorly even vis-à-vis Dalits, which highlights why it is important to focus on individuals in the final analysis. A central focus on both aggregative and individual capabilities is needed—only then would the pursuit of justice be progressive, dynamic and inclusive. It should eventually be about social justice rather than social jealousies, which is a rather primordial way of pursuing justice. As a country moving towards modernity, our pursuit of justice also has to evolve.

Many policy conclusions can be drawn vis-à-vis access to various determinants of child survival, as discussed before. First, while we should focus on *equality of treatment vis-à-vis the differential capabilities of groups and individuals*, a pursuit of equality in the space of determinants is neither empirically nor normatively desirable (positive pursuit), but should not be discriminatory (negative pursuit of justice). From a prescriptive perspective, let me just say that we need medical pluralism so that various groups and individuals have reasonable options available to them—as per the drug regulatory objectives of 'safety, quality, and efficacy'—which they can access and utilize as per their choice, within the limits affordable to a given State. If there are certain interventions about which the government has sufficient evidence to push for, and cannot wait for parents to make a choice, especially in a context of widespread health illiteracy, they should accord priority to population groups based on their respective outcomes—the worse, the higher the priority—when it comes to reaching out to them *proactively* (as happens in the case of door-to-door mass campaigns). However, two things need to be noted here. One, even then, the choice of parents has to be respected, given that we live in a democracy. However, if the State feels that the intervention is absolutely necessary for the survival of a child, being ultimately responsible for it, it should be allowed to undertake coercive measures as well. However, this should be the final recourse when various ways of convincing the parents have failed. The central focus here is on the child rather than the parents—the former lack choices and responsibilities, the latter is secondary at best in this context. Nevertheless, we need to give this issue more thought and I am a bit hesitant to put forward a firm response in this regard, given the biases and vested interests entrenched in the State and society. Two, despite this proactive approach, those who have an advantage vis-à-vis the outcomes should still not be discriminated / treated unequally when they wish to *opportunistically* access health facilities out of choice.

Second, since the space of the intermediate and structural determinants is more secular and involves variables which, if we were to use Rawls's approach to social primary goods, we could argue are those 'that every rational person is presumed to want whatever else he wants' (Rawls 1971: 174), and, therefore, equality in the space of intermediate and structural determinants needs to be pursued *proactively*, irrespective of outcomes, along with what we mentioned under point one here. In any case, these determinants are not only important from the perspective of child survival—education, wealth, public offices, and so on, are important as part of a broader pursuit of justice, even from a capability perspective. This is why it is not easy or feasible to restrict child survival and flourishing to a narrow focus on healthcare—it is influenced by, and has to be part of, the wider practice of justice. Even if one were to accept that the negative goal of bare survival *could* be achieved by neglecting these broader determinants—assuming a high degree of access to and quality of healthcare—the pursuit of justice and equity in the context of the positive goal, of children's flourishing, cannot be achieved by ignoring them. As we argued in Chapter 1, not only are children the worst victims of injustices and inequalities, they offer the best chance to address intergenerational inequalities in opportunities and outcomes. Therefore, there is no reason why we should not make children the central—although not exclusive—focus for all our policies and initiatives related to social justice. This is what we owe our children; this is what justice for children and justice in general should mean. And this is what would set the developing nations particularly on the dynamic path of equity along with aggregative achievement. The thresholds of development in these countries are so low that a static pursuit of equality of the attainment variety would be disastrous for growth as well as flourishing of individuals and groups.

Implications for Political Philosophy

Despite their contextual rootedness, our discussions here have several implications for the political philosophical debates and public policy pursuit of justice. Justice for children seems to encapsulate a broader pursuit of justice, given its interconnections with the status of women and households. In fact, it has the potential to anchor the broader pursuit of justice by being considered as a suitable outcome measure for it—would it matter for parents that they achieve social justice without passing on its benefits to their children, for instance? In other words, given that parents generally try to do the best for their children, when their children are dying or are unable to achieve their flourishing—flourishing is what parents generally try to achieve for their children—it would generally indicate how well their parents, especially mothers, are doing. From this perspective, child mortality could also be broadly considered as one of the important indicators of maternal justice in particular. Child survival should, therefore, be central to theoretical debates as well as the practical pursuit of justice. Children, rather than 'the basic structure of society'—as we argued in the first chapter, contrary to the Rawlsian approach—should be 'the primary subject of justice' (Rawls 1971: 3). A theory of justice focused on humans—especially children, the future of our societies—and their flourishing rather than social, political and economic structures is needed for the pursuit of equity along with growth in developing countries in particular. Many a time, in their eagerness for rapid growth and riddance of evils like poverty, political leaders in developing countries have committed some of the worst injustices against their own citizens—a theory of justice should be able to address the compulsions of growth with equity. Sen's approach seems capable of doing that, while the resourcist ones have the potential to exacerbate a non-human (obviously, not *inhuman*) focus in public policy.

A central focus on children is a central implication of this work for the debates of justice in political philosophy. As highlighted earlier, modern theories of justice ignored children because they have not regarded them as full citizens, capable of choice and responsibility—the latter seen as the most central concept in these theories of justice. Nevertheless, as we saw in the last two chapters, even children's bare survival—let alone their health, flourishing or future prospects in life—is so directly influenced by patterns of injustice. How do we decide on the suitability of an equalisandum without taking into consideration the worst victims of injustice—given that children start out with massive inequities even before they come into the world, without any choice or control over their prospects? From a quantitative perspective as well, how can a theory of justice that ignores more than a quarter of the world population, which children in the age group of 0–14 years are, be considered tenable? On the other hand, one could argue that those metrics of justice that are able to account for various segments of the population have an advantage from an empirical as well as a practical-normative perspective. Theories of justice have to be inclusionary rather than exclusionary in their approach. The same can be said in the context of their applicability to very different contexts and injustices. Sen's metric and approach to justice, for reasons discussed in this and the previous chapters, would score over its competitors as far as these concerns are concerned.

What better can one expect from theories conceptualized in abstraction, divorced from empirical realities? An engagement with the complex everyday life is not even an expectation from political philosophers in the Western world—philosophers studying the 'political' rather than abstract fields like logic or metaphysics, for instance. In most developing countries, on the other hand, there is usually a strong expectation from academics—by funding agencies as well as others—to undertake research with a direct practical relevance, given their developmental challenges and impatience to spend on non-practical—not necessarily impractical though, as we have tried to demonstrate—areas of research. This is probably one of the reasons why political philosophy developed in the Western world, and remained underdeveloped in the developing, in modern times. In ancient times, though, there were illustrious philosophers in the currently developing world as well. Anyway, this is not the right place to dwell on the issue any further. It is, however, important to appreciate that political philosophers need to have, at least, some sort of empirical orientation or adopt the case-implication approach (Sen 1979) more often—or, at least, treat those who do with respect rather than disdain.[13] Non-philosophers, too, should venture

---

[13] See Michael Marmot's *Foreword* in Venkatapuram (2011): 'First, why did this philosopher feel no need to engage with a non-philosopher? Why come to an interdisciplinary meeting if the perspectives of other disciplines were too ill-informed, too worthy of contempt, to be of interest? Second, why did he not think that a real-life problem was of interest—he seemed to be engaged in highly theoretical discussion that engaged not at all with the real world? Third … to dismiss educational differences between socio-economic groups as "probably genetic" was worse than ignorant…. If knowledge of how the real world

into the political philosophers' terrain using this approach, without worrying about being treated with disdain, as bridging of gap between the abstract and the mundane ought to be multidisciplinary—with beginnings, even if not perfect, or to the satisfaction of puritans ruling the disciplinary fortresses. Let political philosophers take offense, and hopefully respond—they would, at least, be drawn down to the mundane, which they, on their own, may not.

Nevertheless, even though Sen's earlier works were extensively empirical in their orientation, his philosophical works, like that of his Western counterparts, have been more abstract than evidence based. And so, like theirs, his philosophical works also need to be put to evidence-based analysis. However, my bigger concern is with the *development*, and not mere application or testing, of theory in the developing world, based on actual injustices that not only negatively affect the opportunities for flourishing of the individuals and groups living in them, but its development prospects at large. Political philosophy, much more than the social sciences, is still caught up in its modern Western paradigm, although Sen did invoke several ancient Asian philosophers in *Idea of Justice* (2009), while Dalit scholars like Gopal Guru have delved into philosophical conceptualizations of justice based on the particular experience of Dalit communities in India as well as generally. We also need to refer to the work done by the highly eminent social anthropologist, André Béteille, in this regard. However, as Rawls said regarding the critics of utilitarianism, 'they failed, I believe, to construct a workable and systematic moral conception to oppose it', a vacuum which he tried to fill through his own monumental *A Theory of Justice* (Rawls 1971: viii). We need works of comparable calibre to emerge from the developing world, albeit grounded in its own peculiar evidence and experience of injustices. The argument for having theories of justice from the developing world as well is not a parochial one, but one aimed at widening and universalizing the horizon of existing discussions so that the injustices that the developing world faces are more adequately reflected at a theoretical level as well as in practical public policies. At the same time, this would also have the potential to make Western theories of justice

---

worked was irrelevant to his philosophy, might the converse be true: that his philosophy was irrelevant to the real world?' This seems to be the case with most political philosophers, including Rawls.

more empirically oriented and relevant than they are now, given the strong empirical focus in the developing world.

As a concluding thought, let me add that individuals around the world, especially in the developing, deserve justice, not just development as traditionally understood by governments and international organizations—focused on the basic provision of resources in the areas of health, education, and so on, as a matter of generosity by State and non-State actors. They deserve optimal flourishing of their potentials rather than bare survival, manageable health and well-being. The dominant development discourse needs a powerful vision based on sound principles of justice so that its bar can be raised and development goals are designed in a way that they reflect the imperative of human flourishing. We urgently need visionaries in policymaking to balance—not to replace—the influence of high-flying technocrats on national and international policymaking. They have and are making a great contribution, but lack vision—political philosophy, if not philosophers, can fill that gap in policy.

Implications for Affirmative Action Policies

Our discussion also has several implications for the general pursuit of justice, which I would like to briefly highlight without elaboration (for rationale, kindly refer to preceding discussions).

In the final run, assessment and pursuit of justice has to be focused on individuals, irrespective of background. However, this does not mean that we should ignore *social* or other forms of aggregate injustices, which are so clearly reflected in accesses and outcomes of a wide variety.

This leads us to our second point. Especially in a country like India where aggregate achievements are poor, the pursuit of justice has to be complex and dynamic so that the concerns of equity and efficiency are simultaneously addressed. In the context of pervasive human diversity, which would probably not be as characteristic of any other country as India, policymakers should focus on the enhancement of *capabilities* of various groups and individuals, and not just those of the worst off. Capability, rather than caste, should be the central focal variable based on which affirmative action policies should be designed—the two overlap in several contexts, but not always. There are cross-cutting axes of deprivation as well that should be taken care of—for example, within Dalits, the position of women and religious groups or various subcastes; within women, the position of Dalit and other women. The ambit of affirmative action has to be broader, on the one hand, and more nuanced, on the other. The definition of worst off also varies with the particular concern and context under consideration. There are innumerable examples in Chapters 3 and 4 that demonstrate how it is not always females, SCs or STs who are the worst performers. In such contexts, should we ignore those who have been historically privileged? We need to consider, but move beyond traditional stereotypical categories.

A complex pursuit of justice should be multidisciplinary, multisectoral, and multifocal in its approach.

References

Arneson, Richard. 2006. 'Distributive Justice and Basic Capability Equality: "Good Enough" is Not Good Enough'. In *Capabilities Equality*, edited by Alexander Kaufman, 17–43. New York: Routledge.

Bhalotra, Sonia, Christine Valente, and Arthur van Soest. 2010. 'Religion and Childhood Death in India'. In *Handbook of Muslims in India*, edited by Rakesh Basant and Abusaleh Shariff, 123–64. New Delhi: Oxford University Press.

CSDH. 2008. *Closing the Gap in a Generation. Health Equity through Action on the Social Determinants of Health (Final report of the Commission on Social Determinants of Health)*. Geneva: World Health Organization.

Haider, Batool and Zulfiqar Bhutta. 2014. 'Neonatal Vitamin A Supplementation: Time to Move on'. *The Lancet* 385(9975): 1268–71.

Kapoor, Soumya, Deepa Narayan, Saumik Paul, and Nina Badgaiyan. 2009. 'Caste Dynamics and Mobility in Uttar Pradesh'. In *Moving out of Poverty*, edited by Deepa Narayan, Lant Pritchett, and Soumya Kapoor, 166–233. Washington, DC: The World Bank and Palgrave Macmillan.

OECD. OECD Family Database. https://stats.oecd.org/Index.aspx?DataSet Code=FAMILY (accessed 25 August 2018).

Pai, Sudha. 2004. 'Dalit Question and Political Response: Comparative Study of Uttar Pradesh and Madhya Pradesh'. *Economic and Political Weekly* 39(11): 1141–50.

Pritchett, Lant and Charles Kenny. 2013. *Promoting Millennium Development Ideals. The Risks of Defining Development Down*. Washington, DC: Center for Global Development (CGDEV).

Rawls, John. 1971. *A Theory of Justice*. Cambridge, MA and London: The Belknap Press of Harvard University Press.

————. 2008. *The Law of Peoples. With 'The Idea of Public Reason Revisited'*. New Delhi: Universal Law Publishing.

Ruger, Jennifer. 2009. *Health and Social Justice*. New York: Oxford University Press.

Sachar Committee Report. 2006. 'Social, Economic and Educational Status of the Muslim Community of India: A Report'. Prime Minister's High Level Committee, Cabinet Secretariat, Government of India.

Sen, Amartya. 1979. *Equality of What?* The Tanner Lecture on Human Values. Stanford: Stanford University.

————. 1995. *Inequality Reexamined*. New York: Russell Sage Foundation; Cambridge, MA: Harvard University Press.

————. 2002. 'Why Health Equity?' *Health Economics* 11(8): 659–66.

————. 2009. *The Idea of Justice*. Cambridge, MA: The Belknap Press of Harvard University Press.

UNICEF. 2017. 'The State of the World's Children 2017 Statistical Tables'. https://data.unicef.org/resources/state-worlds-children-2017-statistical-tables/ (accessed 25 August 2018).

UNPD. 2011. *World Population Prospects*. New York: Department of Economic and Social Affairs (DESA), Population Division.

van de Poel, Ellen, and Niko Speybroeck. 2009. 'Decomposing Malnutrition Inequalities between Scheduled Castes and Tribes and the Remaining Indian Population'. *Ethnicity & Health* 14(3): 271–87.

Venkatapuram, Sridhar. 2011. *Health Justice: An Argument from the Capabilities Approach*. Cambridge: Polity Press.

Williams, Alan. 1997. 'Intergenerational Equity: An Exploration of the "Fair Innings" Argument'. *Health Economics* 6(2): 117–32.

World Bank. 2004. 'Attaining the Millennium Development Goals in India: How Likely and What Will It Take to Reduce Infant Mortality, Child Malnutrition, Gender Disparities and Hunger-Poverty and to Increase School Enrollment and Completion?'. Report No. 30266-IN, Human Development Unit, South Asia Region, The World Bank, Washington, DC.

Index

About the Author

Ali Mehdi is a senior fellow at the Indian Council for Research on International Economic Relations (ICRIER), a premier Indian policy research institution. He established the *Health Policy Initiative* at ICRIER in 2014 and has been leading it since.

Mehdi has more than 13 years of experience in health research—on themes ranging from health equity and justice to chronic diseases, drug regulation and antimicrobial resistance. He was part of G20 health discussions and policy brief in 2017, and co-authored a report for India's Ministry of Finance for its health engagement at the G20 in 2018. Among his other recent works are: a forthcoming edited volume tentatively titled, *Health of the Nation: India Health Report* (Oxford University Press 2019) and a co-authored book, *Freedoms, fragility and job creation: Perspectives from Jammu and Kashmir, India* (Springer 2018).

Mehdi completed his Master's Degree from Albert-Ludwigs Universität Freiburg and Doctorate from Humboldt-Universität zu Berlin, both in Germany.